612.2 New

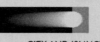
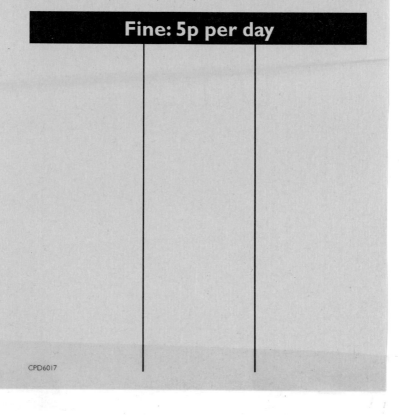

City and Islington Sixth Form College
The Angel 283-309 Goswell Road
London EC1V 7LA
020 7520 0652

CITY AND ISLINGTON
COLLEGE

This book is due for return on or before the date last stamped below.
You may renew by telephone. Please quote the Barcode No.
May not be renewed if required by another reader.

Fine: 5p per day

CPD6017

THE NEW

Severe Acute Respiratory Syndrome

GL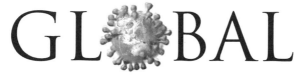BAL

And Its Impacts

THREAT

Editors

Prof Tommy Koh
Director, Institute of Policy Studies, Singapore
and
Ambassador-at-large

Prof Aileen Plant
Professor of International Health
Curtin University of Technology, Australia

Prof Eng Hin Lee
Director, Division of Graduate Medical Studies
and formerly
Dean of Faculty of Medicine, National University of Singapore

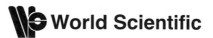 **World Scientific**

NEW JERSEY • LONDON • SINGAPORE • SHANGHAI • HONG KONG • TAIPEI • BANGALORE

Published by

World Scientific Publishing Co. Pte. Ltd.

5 Toh Tuck Link, Singapore 596224

USA office: Suite 202, 1060 Main Street, River Edge, NJ 07661

UK office: 57 Shelton Street, Covent Garden, London WC2H 9HE

British Library Cataloguing-in-Publication Data
A catalogue record for this book is available from the British Library.

CITY AND ISLINGTON
SIXTH FORM COLLEGE
283 - 309 GOSWELL ROAD
LONDON
EC1
TEL 020 7520 0652

THE NEW GLOBAL THREAT
Severe Acute Respiratory Syndrome and Its Impacts

ISBN 981-238-665-3
ISBN 981-238-668-8 (pbk)

Printed in Singapore by Mainland Press

Contents

Editorial by Professor Tommy Koh   vii

Editorial by Professor Aileen J. Plant   xiii

Editorial by Professor Eng Hin Lee   xxv

Section I: WHO: Role and Influence

1.   WHO: At the Forefront of Combating SARS   3

Section II: China

2.   Fighting Infectious Diseases: One Mission, Many Agents   17
   Shiping Tang

3.   SARS, Anti-Populism, and Elite Lies: Temporary
   Disorders in China   31
   Lynn T. White III

4.   Baptism by Storm: The SARS Crisis' Imprint on China's
   New Leadership   69
   Christopher A. McNally

Section III: Hong Kong

5.   The Impact of SARS on Hong Kong Society and Culture:
   Some Personal Reflections   93
   Leo Ou-fan Lee

6.   SARS and the HKSAR Governing Crisis   107
   Ma Ngok

7.   The Social Impact of SARS: Sustainable Action for the
   Rejuvenation of Society   123
   Cecilia L.W. Chan

8.   Catching SARS in the HKSAR: Fallout on Economy
   and Community   147
   Yun-Wing Sung and Fanny M. Cheung

9.   Will SARS Result in a Financial Crisis? —Differentiating
     Real, Transient, and Permanent Economic Effects of a
     Health Crisis   165
     Frank T. Lorne

10. Facing the Unknowns of SARS in Hong Kong   173
     Kwok-yung Yuen and Malik Peiris

Section IV: Singapore

11. Sars, Policy-making and Lesson-drawing   195
     Khai Leong Ho

12. SARS: A Psychological Perspective   209
     George D. Bishop

13. Cracking the Genome of the SARS Virus   221
     Lawrence W. Stanton

14. The Infection Control Response to SARS in Hospitals
     and Institutions   243
     Paul A. Tambyah

15. SARS — Lessons on the Role of Social Responsibility in
     Containing an Epidemic   273
     Pheng-Soon Lee

16. Combating SARS with Infrared Fever Screening System (IFss)   283
     Yang How Tan

Section V: Taiwan

17. Epidemiology and Control of Severe Acute Respiratory
     Syndrome (SARS) Outbreak in Taiwan   301
     Chien-Jen Chen, Yin-Chu Chien and Hwai-I Yang

Section VI: Toronto

18. SARS in Canada: The Story of SARS in Canada is Essentially
     Toronto's Tale   317
     Pauline Chan

EDITORIAL

by TOMMY KOH

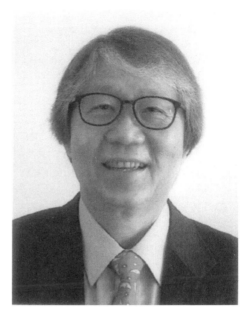

A nation, like an individual, is tested by crisis. A crisis could break a nation, revealing all its weaknesses and negative characteristics. On the other hand, a nation could emerge stronger from a crisis. Singapore emerged stronger from the SARS crisis. The government made some mistakes initially. It was, however, quick to change, in the light of new information and experience. The people responded very well, with the doctors, nurses and other healthcare workers showing courage, commitment and grace under enormous stress. The bond between the government and the people became stronger. It reminded me of the exemplary manner in which the New Yorkers coped with the tragedy of 11 September 2001. What lessons have I learned from the way in which Singapore has overcome the SARS crisis?

First, the Singapore Government, unlike some other governments, did not deny that Singapore had patients suffering from SARS. It is an unfortunate fact that some governments try to deny bad news. The lesson I have learned is that is it counter-productive for governments to be in a denial mode. It is better to face the facts.

Second, it is better to be transparent than to be opaque. Some governments tried to take refuge by not telling its own people, the WHO and the media what the facts were. The Singapore government was wise in deciding, from the start of the crisis, to tell the news, both good and bad, in a calm and factual way, to the people everyday. The timely delivery of information to the people helps to instil confidence. The absence of such information prompts a people to indulge in speculation and to depend on hear-say. Transparency is a better public policy than opacity.

Third, in order to make the right policy one must make a thorough study of the nature of the crisis. The Singapore government mobilized all available resources, both domestic and foreign, to understand the nature of the coronavirus which caused the disease, how it is spread, how it can be contained, and how to help patients recover from the disease. The Singaporean team of doctors, virologists, geneticists, public health and communicable diseases specialists, and other experts was aided in their tasks by experts from the WHO and the Centers for Disease Control of the United States.

Fourth, the Singapore government decided to designate one hospital, the Tan Tock Seng Hospital as the SARS hospital. The doctors, nurses and other healthcare workers of that hospital rose to the challenge. There was no panic in the hospital. The hospital did not have to lock its doors in order to prevent its doctors, nurses and other health workers from fleeing from danger. On the contrary, doctors and nurses from other hospitals volunteered to work at Tan Tock Seng. The heroism of the doctors, nurses and other healthcare workers inspired the whole nation. In retrospect, one can say that the designation of Tan Tock Seng as the SARS hospital was the right decision.

Fifth, the Singapore government decided to trace every person who had been in contact with a SARS patient. This was no easy task in spite of Singapore's small size. The government had to mobilize the human and technological resources of the police, army, People's Association, etc. to this end. Given the manner in which the disease was spread, the decision to trace every contact, no matter how many and how difficult was clearly a right decision.

Sixth, the Singapore government decided to impose home quarantine on persons who had come into contact with a SARS patient who had no symptoms of the disease. This was necessary because an infected person may develop symptoms of the disease and become infectious within a ten-day incubation period. Parliament had to rush through a law to authorize home quarantine and to punish those who violated it. Public opinion had to be mobilized to support an action which was both coercive and intrusive. Cameras, linked to computers, were installed in the homes of persons who were subject to home quarantine orders. On the whole, Singaporeans accepted the need for such measures and responded well. There were many examples of neighbors who went out of their way to help other neighbors who were unable to leave their homes because they were subject to home quarantine orders.

Seventh, the people of Singapore responded to the crisis in an extraordinary way. Many citizens came forward as volunteers, to man counters, to measure temperatures, to set up websites, to man call centers, to deliver food to people under home quarantine orders, etc. The Singapore Chinese Orchestra went to the Tan Tock Seng Hospital to perform in order to cheer up the healthcare workers.

Eighth, new technology, in the form of thermal scanners, were developed or imported and installed at the airport, the causeway, and many other public places. The lesson here is that in fighting a crisis such as this, a multi-disciplinary approach is necessary. There must be no artificial boundary between medicine and engineering or between medicine and other disciplines.

Ninth, the government, the private sector and civil society joined hands in waging a campaign to raise the standards of personal and public hygiene, to take one's temperature daily, to wash one hands thoroughly, and to avoid certain bad habits. The campaign was successfully executed.

Tenth, Singapore was conscious of her responsibility not to export the disease. It therefore implemented measures at our border checkpoints in order to make sure that we detect incoming passengers and visitors with SARS symptoms and send them for screening. We also screened our outgoing passengers in order to prevent the export of the disease.

In conclusion, I would say that of the countries and territories in Asia which were affected by the SARS crisis, Hanoi probably performed best. Singapore probably deserves the second prize. The Singapore SARS story is worth recording because it is a defining moment in Singapore's history and because it is a good case study for students of public policy and crisis management.

TOMMY KOH

Professor Tommy Koh is currently Ambassador-At-Large at the Ministry of Foreign Affairs; Director, Institute of Policy Studies and Chairman of the National Heritage Board. He is also a Director of SingTel and Chairman of the Chinese Heritage Centre.

Prof Koh was the Dean of the Faculty of Law of the University of Singapore from 1971 to 1974. He was Singapore's Permanent Representative to the United Nations, New York from 1968 to 1971 (concurrently accredited as High Commissioner to Canada) and again from 1974 to 1984 (concurrently accredited as High Commissioner to Canada and Ambassador to Mexico). He was Ambassador to the United States of America from 1984 to 1990. He was President of the Third UN Conference on the Law of the Sea from 1980 to 1982. He was Chairman of the Preparatory Committee and the Main Committee of the UN Conference on Environment and Development from 1990 to 1992. He was the founding Chairman of the National Arts Council from 1991 to 1996 and Director of the Institute of Policy Studies from 1990 to February 1997. From February 1997 to October 2000, he served as the founding Executive Director of the Asia-Europe Foundation. He is also Singapore's Chief Negotiator for the US-Singapore Free Trade Agreement (2000 to 2003).

Prof Koh was appointed by the United Nations Secretary-General as his Special Envoy to lead a mission to the Russian Federation, Latvia, Lithuania and Estonia in August/September 1993. Prof Koh was a member of three WTO dispute panels, two of which as Chairman.

Prof Koh was the Second Arthur & Frank Payne Visiting Professor at the Institute for International Studies, Stanford University, USA, for 1994/95. He is a visiting Professor at Zhejiang University. Prof Koh is on the Board of Directors of the Institute for the Study of Diplomacy at Georgetown University. He is a member of the International Council of The Asia Society (New York) and a co-convenor of its Williamsburg Conference. He is also a member of the International Advisory Committee of the Korean Federation of Industries.

Prof Koh received a First Class Honours degree in Law from the National University of Singapore, has a Masters degree in Law from Harvard University and a post-graduate Diploma in Criminology from Cambridge University.

He was conferred a full professorship in 1977. In 1984, Prof Koh was awarded an Honorary Degree of Doctor of Laws from Yale University. He has also received awards from Columbia University, Stanford University, Georgetown University, the Fletcher School of Law and Diplomacy and Curtin University. On 22 September 2002, Prof Koh was conferred an Honorary Degree of Doctor of Laws from Monash University.

For his service to the nation, Prof Koh was awarded the Public Service Star in 1971, the Meritorious Service Medal in 1979 and the Distinguished Service Order Award in 1990. Prof Koh was appointed Commander in the Order of the Golden Ark by HRH Prince Bernhard of the Netherlands in March 1993. He received the award of the Grand Cross of the Order of Bernardo O'Higgins from the Government of Chile on 3 April 1997. He also received the 1996 Elizabeth Haub Prize from the University of Brussels and the International Council on Environmental Law on 17 April 1997. Prof Koh was awarded the 1998 Fok Ying Tung Southeast Asia Prize by the Fok Ying Tung Foundation in Hong Kong on 29 May 1998. On 22 February 2000 he was awarded the "Commander, First Class, of the Order of the Lion of Finland" by the President of Finland. On 2 May 2000, he was conferred the title of "Grand Officer in the Order of Merit of the Grand Duchy of Luxembourg" by the Prime Minister of Luxembourg. On 6 August 2001, he was conferred the rank of Officer in the Order of the Legion of Honour by the President of the French Republic. Presented with the Peace and Commerce Award by the US Secretary of Commerce, Donald Evans, in Washington DC, on 5 May 2003.

[August 2003]

Editorial

SARS and Public Health: Lessons for Future Epidemics

by *AILEEN J. PLANT*

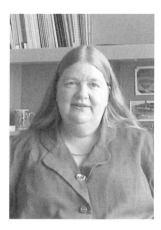

An unknown disease that spreads rapidly between countries and for which there is neither prevention in the form of vaccine nor curative drugs seems more like science fiction or a nightmare than reality, and yet in some ways it is exactly this pandemic scenario that public health practitioners have been predicting. The advent of Severe Acute Respiratory Syndrome (SARS) could have been the pandemic of influenza, or a terrorist event. The issues surrounding the response and management are very similar from the perspective of public health management.

It is not many decades ago that in all countries there was an extensive infrastructure devoted to the control of infectious diseases. As most infectious diseases are prevented by good living standards (e.g. adequate food and nutrition, non-crowded living and working conditions and the ready availability of basic healthcare), the emphasis has shifted to more chronic causes of ill-health and death. Increasingly, disease can be prevented by behavior change rather than by laws. Of course, in most countries, laws still play a major role in the appropriate protection of health. Such laws include governance around proper provision of food and water, proper disposal of waste, the unacceptability of spreading certain diseases (and the potential to detain those individuals who do not comply with these standards), and so on. Most countries have some provisions for the notification of specified diseases.

In the last 2–3 decades, we have witnessed approximately one new disease occurring each year, including AIDS, variant Creutzfeldt-Jacob disease, Nipah virus disease to name but three. Most of the 20–30 new diseases have not caused global problems, although of course, AIDS is one disease that has had a major global impact. The reasons for non-impact are varied but include inefficient means of transmission, non-sustainability in human hosts and rapid public health actions. At the same time, there has been a resurgence of some diseases that were previously thought to be declining, such as tuberculosis and malaria. Regardless of the actual disease, public health practitioners fear the advent of a new or resurgent disease that will spread readily between people, and have a significant mortality. Of course, a deliberate release of a biological agent could come under this category.

The changing global situation, as well as the developments in communication technology, computers, and laboratory expertise, all have an impact on how we identify, diagnose, control and monitor diseases.

In this article, I aim to focus on the public health aspects of the control of international outbreaks, using SARS as an example, and including lessons for future outbreaks.

The Current Situation with Outbreaks of International Significance

Currently, outbreaks which are considered to be of international importance are identified, verified and if necessary, external assistance is provided by the World Health Organization (WHO). There is no compulsion on a country to notify diseases other than plague, yellow fever or cholera, and no compulsion for a country to answer truthfully (or even answer) questions as to whether an event is occurring, regardless of the implications of the event for other countries.

An outbreak of international concern is one that is serious, plus of unknown, unusual or possibly not of natural origin. As well, a disease crossing borders between countries or having the potential to cross borders clearly makes a disease of international concern. Lastly, the potential for a disease to have an impact on travel or trade, possibly leading to sanctions, is also of international concern. Perhaps the best way of thinking of whether a disease is of international concern is 'if our neighbor had this disease and we didn't, would we want to know?' There are distinctions between the international (versus the national) importance of a disease.

In the last decade, WHO has established the 'Outbreak Verification List" in which it collects information from a number of sources, including its regional and country offices, country governments and the media about postulated outbreaks. It then confirms that an event exists (i.e., it is not just a rumor) even if the actual diagnosis is unclear, and posts the existence of an outbreak to the List, while offering help for investigation and response. The event remains on the List until the outbreak is either stable or resolved. The List is circulated to a wide number of public health professionals around the world on a confidential basis. WHO does not publicly announce that a country has a disease unless the individual country confirms the validity of the information and agrees that the information is available to the public. Despite these limitations, in recent years knowledge that outbreaks are occurring in various countries has improved greatly, at least in part because of the extraordinary impact of communication technology.

What happens when a country requests assistance? The majority of help provided to countries is advice regarding laboratory expertise, sources of drugs and supplies and so on; however, WHO may dispatch vaccines or antibiotics or even, in comparatively uncommon instances, dispatch a team to assist countries to deal with an outbreak. WHO may raise funds to support the provision of supplies or link the country with specific expertise. Of particular significance is that WHO supports the Global Outbreak and Alert Response Network (GOARN), which is a global network of institutions and people ready to respond to outbreaks when they occur. For instance, an outbreak of Ebola may lead to a request for assistance which will be transmitted to GOARN via email, with a request, for example for a clinician, two epidemiologists and a medical anthropologist. Individuals will respond and attend the outbreak to assist local ministries of health, but operate under the WHO mandate. This means that there is a large and diverse group of people available to assist in a whole range of scenarios, without the need for a large army on continual standby for what are (generally) occasional events. For instance, this occurred in SARS when the WHO Office in Vietnam requested assistance and an email was sent to GOARN members looking for people prepared to go to Vietnam.

Of course, none of this precludes bilateral assistance such as often occurs. For instance, Canada did not ask WHO for assistance in dealing with its SARS outbreak but asked the US for assistance and a team from CDC, Atlanta was dispatched to assist the Canadian health department.

However, at the moment, all the collaboration between countries and WHO is done on the basis of goodwill, and there are no formal agreements about dealing with outbreaks apart from the requirement under the International Health Regulations to notify plague, cholera and yellow fever, regardless of how much threat a disease may pose for other countries. WHO cannot, under the current arrangements, oblige a country to respond to queries about events even if such an event is a major risk to nearby countries.

Particular Issues in the International Spread of Disease

In the world of today, diseases spread faster and have a greater (or at least faster) impact on global economies than in previous centuries. The issues surrounding travel and trade are immense. At the same time, the processes of trade and travel are becoming more globalized, so the potential for disease being spread inadvertently is greater than ever. For SARS, people who were later found to be carrying the SARS virus had traveled from Hong Kong to many countries including Vietnam, Singapore, and Canada, from where they spread the disease to many others within those countries. However, we could not stop people (or goods) traveling in case they later are found to be carrying a deadly disease, without the complete halt of all travel and trade.

In these days of global markets, countries are dependent on trade. The process of industrialization has led to a mutual inter-dependence, whereby each country is dependent on others for their economic survival. A disease that affects travel and trade can effectively rip an enormous amount out of the national budget and may even send whole businesses bankrupt. We certainly have seen the impact on trade of several diseases, such as the plague in India in 1994; bovine spongiform encephalopathy or so-called "mad cow disease" and its human equivalent, Creutzfeldt-Jacob Syndrome in the United Kingdom; and more recently the impact on Canada's beef trade of the first BSE-contaminated herd. The real challenge is to balance the protection of human health with the protection of trade, without letting either become such a dominant force that the other is compromised. Many diseases have an inevitable economic effect which translates back to an effect on health, far greater than the impact of the disease itself. The impact of the plague in India affected a relatively small number of individuals, and while for these individuals, plague was a tragedy, the real impact of plague was felt by those people who became poverty stricken and unable to access even the most basic necessities of life when two billion US dollars was lost as a result of international actions because of fears about plague.

The most recent disease having a global impact on travel, trade and their associated economies is, of course, SARS. The impact of SARS on the economies of Asia is still being calculated. What will be much harder to work out is the impact of these economic insults on health.

The SARS Outbreak in Vietnam

The outbreak in Vietnam was the first documentation of what we now call SARS, even though we now believe that the disease first arose in southern China. SARS in Vietnam began when a Chinese-American businessman was admitted to a small private-for-profit hospital in Hanoi on the 26 February. WHO in Vietnam was advised early because the man had been in southern China and then Hong Kong, and local doctors were concerned that he had influenza. At approximately the same time, a couple of cases of "bird flu" had been diagnosed in Hong Kong that were of concern, hence the contact with WHO. On the 5 February, six healthcare workers were admitted to hospital with a similar infection to that of the first man. The same day, the index case was evacuated to Hong Kong, where he died a week later. WHO requested and was granted a meeting with senior ministry officials on the weekend of the 8 and 9 of March, and it is to the credit of the Vice-Minister for Health and the Minister for Health that the WHO advice regarding the emergency and the need for external assistance was agreed. It required considerable leadership to act in these difficult circumstances. The speed with which action occurred still remains the fastest of any government to the best of my knowledge.

Within 24 hours infectious disease epidemiologists were en route to Hanoi, and by the time the outbreak was over, a huge local team plus a total of 24 foreigners had participated as part of the SARS response.

Dr. Carlo Urbani, a WHO employee saw the first and subsequent cases and provided the world's first description of what we now know as SARS. By the 11 March, he too developed symptoms and was dead by the end of the month.

In Vietnam, the Prime Minister established an intersectoral SARS committee, demonstrating leadership across government and by doing so supporting the Minister for Health in her efforts to control SARS.

In all, 63 epidemiologically linked SARS cases were associated with one index case. The attack rate for clinical SARS disease varied from 30% among hospital workers with patient-contact, 6.5% among patients hospitalized for other diseases at one hospital, and 6.3% among close contacts of one case. At least 4 generations of transmission were identified. Including 3 cases that were exported to other countries, the overall case fatality was 10.9%.

These figures do not convey the fear, heartbreak, courage and commitment that were demonstrated throughout the outbreak. The workers of the French Hospital went through a horrendous experience where about one in every five workers at the hospital came down with SARS. Even having been in Vietnam at the time I cannot imagine going to work every day, continuing to look after your colleagues and then feeling the beginnings of this new disease in yourself, not knowing at that time whether everyone who got the disease would die. And yet, in Vietnam, I do not know of anyone who ran away, who refused to do their job because of personal fears. Some were stigmatized and not allowed home, some did not want to go home because of the fear of infecting their families. The net effect was that the hospital became partially quarantined from the rest of the community, as doctors and nurses probably infected each other more frequently than other people outside the hospital.

Later, the private hospital stopped accepting new patients (except for their own staff who became ill with SARS), and a public hospital was designated the SARS hospital. Intensive effort was put into surveillance, contact tracing and infection control. Major effort was required to maintain media liaison, educate health workers and the public throughout the country, and to ensure the ready supply of goods needed for proper infection control.

On the 28 April, the outbreak was declared to be contained by the Minister of Health for Vietnam, the first country in the world to do so. As in all countries, infection control, surveillance and response had to be upgraded; from each country there are many lessons for both dealing with SARS and for preparing for the next outbreak that will inevitably arise.

Some of the Lessons from SARS

Many lessons were learnt from SARS. Two I have already alluded to: the importance of speed and leadership. Without speed, the number of people infected or potentially infected with SARS increases rapidly, both increasing the chance that the disease will get out of control and putting excessive strain on the health services. Because of the impact of SARS on travel and trade, leadership is necessary if the appropriate actions are to be undertaken. This means that leadership has to be at a high enough level in government for a whole-of-government approach — for instance, the establishment of an intersectoral committee. Such intersectoral committees are essential, and will probably need to meet daily at the height of an outbreak.

The SARS response (or any response to an infectious disease) needs to take into account the existing health structures and work with them as much as possible, ensuring that there is a clear chain of command. This is an important factor if the response is to be sustainable and to have local credibility.

Technical assistance is essential in most outbreaks — the knowledge base around managing and investigating outbreaks is complex and demanding, and requires dedicated personnel. Many countries have established Field Epidemiology Training Programs which provide a core capacity to investigate outbreaks. Graduates of many of these programs were exceptionally valuable in the SARS response. Existing infrastructure and systems that are available and functioning in areas of surveillance and response will permit rapid action and early action in the case of new diseases.

In the cases of SARS, issues surrounding infection control were of paramount importance. Because every case potentially infects others, isolation in order that no further people can be infected is essential if the chain of transmission is to be broken. We know (now) that maximum infectiousness in SARS is late, compared with many other infectious diseases, so contact tracing is especially effective. People do not appear to be infectious prior to the onset of symptoms and it is not until they have had symptoms for about 10 days that they reach maximum infectiousness. This provides an important opportunity to identify contacts and contact them every day to ensure that they are well and have no symptoms. If they become symptomatic they should be isolated, with careful attention to three main risks:

1. that they don't infect others;
2. that until the diagnosis is probable SARS that they don't catch SARS — in case the diagnosis is something else, it is essential that SARS is not spread among those who may have another diagnosis.
3. that appropriate investigation (and treatment) occurs for other possible diagnoses.

All of this pre-supposes that conditions are such that appropriate infection control can be established and maintained; this puts unexpected stresses on even sophisticated hospitals. For other diseases where the main mechanism of spread is airborne such as influenza, it is very unlikely that most hospitals could maintain adequate infection control except for very short periods.

Three other main areas require particular attention in outbreak response such as occurred with SARS: the media, training/education and logistics.

The media have a legitimate interest and an important role in educating and informing the public. However, their demands can overwhelm all available resources, and this means that the media response needs to be planned and managed appropriately. The interaction with the media needs to be timely, transparent and regular. A well-informed public can minimize the economic impact as well as acting as information sources for further cases.

Training and education of all relevant staff and the public is essential. Every hospital in the world that dealt with SARS had to improve their infection control and of course this meant educating every doctor and every nurse. This is particularly important as every individual thinks they already know about infection control, and hence introducing different systems and procedures can be met with a range of attitudes, including outright hostility and defiance. It is essential that a standard of care is set and then mechanisms are in place to ensure that everyone implements such standards. The best way of doing this is to identify as few places as geographically possible (and preferably only one place) for the treatment of SARS, and ensuring good standards are maintained at the one place.

The logistics are often underestimated in dealing with any outbreak; however, in SARS it is essential to ensure that appropriate materials are well-supplied wherever and whenever they are needed. For instance, in Vietnam we found that limited handwashing capacity meant that alcohol-based hand washes were essential and that this did not just mean one-off provision but installation of dispensers and daily attention to whether the containers were being maintained. If good supplies are not maintained, the net result will be the people lowest in the organizational hierarchy are those least likely to have access to the protective equipment, yet most likely to be in direct contact with the infectious patients.

Appropriate use of quarantine (i.e., measures applying to people entering a country) may need to be considered, and possibly the poorer or less infrastructure within a country, the more appropriate quarantine may be. Quarantine will never be perfect but it can decrease the chances of spreading a disease while other systems (such as border screening, surveillance and infection control) are put in place. Quarantine measures should be seen as temporary and as just one of a raft of possible measures.

Separate from quarantine, most governments will also need (or already have) legal powers to detain individuals, and to compel isolation for those few individuals who persist in putting others at risk.

What is Needed for Future Prevention Measures and Programs?

No-one knows where SARS came from, although it is postulated that SARS arose from wild animals. The reasons that this is considered to be true are that animals have been found to be infected with Coronavirus, the etiological cause of SARS, and wild-animal handlers have antibodies to Coronavirus. However, neither of these facts is sufficient to be sure where SARS originated. Without this knowledge, it is difficult to know whether SARS will come back. What is certain, however, is regardless of whether SARS returns, some other infectious disease will occur to challenge governments and health professionals — our challenge is how best to be prepared for such an event.

Future prevention of SARS and similar diseases depends on public health preparedness. Vaccines are unlikely to provide a rapid solution to new diseases unless, of course, they are merely variations of old diseases. By this I mean that it is extremely difficult to tailor-make a safe and effective vaccine at an affordable price in the time-frame of new diseases. We don't have to look very far to see the truth of this — AIDS, hepatitis C, West Nile virus, Nipah virus, Ebola virus to name just a few diseases, that have captured headlines in the last two decades, and for which there are still no vaccines available.

To control diseases we already know about, we need to be able to identify, diagnose and investigate them. The same is true for the diseases that we don't yet know about. This means good scientific capacity, laboratory skills and a developed health system with surveillance and response capacity. It means that the underlying infrastructure has to be in place before diseases, such as SARS, even occurs. It was these skills and infrastructure that permitted the rapid identification and control of SARS, even in the absence of vaccines or specific treatments. And in some instances, it was the lack of existing infrastructure that hampered efforts to control SARS.

The purpose of both the current and the proposed International Health Regulations is to "ensure the maximum security against the international spread of disease with a minimum interference with world traffic." Currently, only cholera, plague and yellow fever are notified to the World Health Organization, and notification is variably implemented. The current regulations are increasingly inappropriate in a world where an individual incubating a disease can be anywhere on the globe within 24 hours, and where traded goods are moved nearly as fast within trading systems that are more open than ever before known.

The current proposal for the revision of the International Health Regulations will require countries to notify WHO if they have "events of international public health significance", and as such has (potentially) a huge role to play. As part of the proposed system, WHO will require a 24-hour a day focal point within each country for communication, as well as the capacity to identify events of concern for notification or to respond to requests for information if concerns are raised by other countries. To some extent the global community, via country endorsement of proposed actions by WHO, has already agreed to share information, to respond appropriately and generally to work together in identifying and controlling disease. The required changes for the revised IHR are being developed now, and it is proposed that the necessary endorsements will be put to the 2005 World Health Assembly. They will provide a way whereby countries can work together to protect public health and a mechanism whereby international pressure can maintain good practice.

Within countries, governments should ensure they have the necessary legal power to know and act accordingly for disease control, while at the same time safeguarding the rights of individuals. This may involve powers around notification of disease, identification of contacts and in rare instances, detention of individuals.

Conclusion

Speed and leadership are the two most important factors to ensure control of an infectious disease such as SARS. Recognizing the impact of outbreaks of diseases also highlights the importance of the non-health sector, especially those sectors concerned with legal issues, tourism, trade and finance. Governments must have sufficient legal power to protect and monitor public health. Within the health sector, it is essential that all appropriate sections are included in preparing for the response, including clinical, diagnostic, surveillance, laboratory, response, media, education and logistics areas.

In the end, SARS was a primarily hospital-acquired infection with limited spread to family and community contacts, that was controlled by old-fashioned contagion control, i.e., the identification and isolation of cases, documentation and follow-up of contacts with immediate isolation should a contact develop any possible SARS-associated symptoms, thereby preventing any further spread of the disease. Although it challenged our capacity to respond, to work together and to implement appropriate action, it was easy compared with what we might have seen if it had been an air-borne disease. SARS was comparatively easy to control, next time we might not be so lucky, and we should learn from the experience.

AILEEN J. PLANT

Dr. Aileen Plant is Professor of International Health at the Curtin University of Technology in Perth and a key player in the recently established Australian Biosecurity Cooperative Research Centre for Emerging Infectious Diseases. She has extensive experience in outbreak investigation and was recently the Coordinator for the World Health Organization SARS Team in Vietnam.

She is a medical graduate of The University of Western Australia, has a Master of Public Health and a PhD from The University of Sydney and a Diploma of Tropical Medicine and Hygiene from London. She is a specialist public health physician and has published 70 peer-reviewed articles as well as writing numerous reports and chapters in books.

She has particular interests in infectious disease epidemiology and control, including surveillance, outbreak investigation, and the interface between research, policy and implementation.

Prior to the SARS outbreak, and during the last 15 years she has worked at WHO for two periods of several months, been the Director of Australia's Field Epidemiology Program at the Australian National University and been Chief Health Officer/Deputy Secretary of the Northern Territory Department of Health. She continues to serve on a range of national and state committees, including the Communicable Disease Network, Australia and Australia's Infectious Disease Emergency Response Committee.

Editorial

The SARS Outbreak — A Nation Rises to the Challenge

by *ENG HIN LEE*

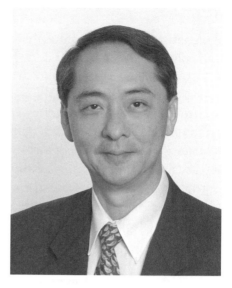

When a new virus such as the one responsible for SARS emerges, seemingly out of nowhere, it often takes us by surprise. Once the virus arrived in the city of Hong Kong, it rapidly spread to other parts of Asia and beyond, aided along by the ease of international air travel. It arrived in Singapore in early March and very quickly wrought havoc in the medical community, claiming the lives of many healthcare workers. Presented with such a deadly disease, the hospitals had to act quickly and decisively to contain the situation.

As it was a new disease, little was known of the causative agent and its habits and characteristics. Learning from the limited experience of the affected countries, we quickly ascertained that the most effective means of preventing infection by the virus was through the use of proper and effective protective gear and the use of barrier nursing techniques. An extensive and comprehensive education program was immediately put in place by all hospitals to train all levels of staff the correct method of hand washing, donning and removal of gloves and gowns, and every single person was tested for proper fit of the N95 mask. Especially vulnerable were the healthcare workers in the Intensive Care Unit, Emergency Department and the medical wards dealing with patients with fever and chest infections. Strict rules regarding the use of Personal Protective Equipment (PPE) were introduced and enforced. Isolation wards were created for patients with fever and Tan Tock Seng Hospital was designated a SARS hospital so that all probable SARS cases could be isolated and contained in one hospital.

At the same time, the Ministry of Health started a nation-wide public education program to inform the community of the seriousness of the situation and to create a high level of awareness and knowledge of the presenting symptoms so that early medical screening and treatment could be instituted. The media helped tremendously in this effort through responsible reporting after each daily press briefing held by the Ministry of Health. Medical experts, especially those in infectious diseases, respiratory diseases and epidemiology from across the nation were called upon to help the administrators in the Ministry of Health and the Hospital Clusters to formulate a plan of action. Index cases had to be identified and contacts traced by a huge force of volunteers and workers. No stone was left unturned to ensure that every single contact was found and screened. Quarantine procedures were put in place. The Infectious Disease Act, which was initially introduced during the times when tuberculosis was rampant, was now evoked and modified so that the quarantine would be more effective. On the other hand, quarantine was also made more palatable by providing stipends to self-employed individuals who had to stay away from their work or business for the mandatory ten days. "What is your temperature today?" became a standard greeting instead of "Good morning" or "How are you?" as daily temperature taking became a routine for everyone. Free thermometers were distributed to school children, workers and even to homes to encourage full participation in this exercise. To prevent further entry and export of SARS, checks were made at all entry and exit points to the country whether by land, sea or air. Temperature scanners were erected in the airport for mass detection of travelers with fever.

As with any new disease, before a cure can be found, the causative agent needs to be identified and fully characterized in terms of its habits and modes of spread. The scientific community responded swiftly and the SARS virus was identified as a member of the coronavirus family by different teams in Singapore, Hong Kong and other affected countries. Knowing what the virus is, of course, not enough. The scientists and doctors proceeded to sequence its genome so that more accurate diagnostic tests could be made. Epidemiologists studied its habits and mode of spread and advised on the proper implementation of preventive measures. Scientists and doctors shared information and materials and formed collaborations so that the research could move ahead more quickly and efficiently. Currently diagnostic tests have been developed and are undergoing evaluation and refinement. Researchers are also working on longer term goals, such as a search for methods of prevention, e.g., the development of vaccines, as well as more specific treatment modalities for the infected patient.

The SARS outbreak has had an enormous impact on life in general. Over the last few months, people avoided going to enclosed public places as large group gatherings were discouraged. At one point, schools were closed for a brief period. Medical students were taken off the wards and continuing education programs for doctors were suspended. Many people stopped shaking hands when they met. Apart from affecting our daily routine, the impact on the economy was far reaching. The greatest impact was felt in the travel and hospitality industry as travelers canceled their business or holiday travel plans. Restaurants and retail shops saw a tremendous decline in business. Large international conferences were canceled or postponed, resulting in huge losses to those involved in the organization of such events.

On a more positive note, SARS has taught us a lot. It has brought the whole nation together to fight a common battle. It has taught us not to take things for granted and to be always prepared for all eventualities. Hospital workers have to be ever vigilant and take appropriate precautionary measures when looking after patients with fever and infections. Heroes and heroines have emerged, with the healthcare workers getting the most accolades for their bravery and resolve in fighting this deadly disease. They have won the respect of the whole nation. Leaders in government and hospitals have managed the situation well and deserve to be commended. And of course everyone in the community has also played his/her part in this battle which has now taken us off the WHO SARS affected list. The generosity of the public has been exemplified by their contributions to the "Courage Fund" which will be used to help victims and the families of this disease.

Things are now returning to normal and there has been a noticeable increase in the patronage of restaurants, cinemas and shopping centers. Air travel has picked up and hotel occupancy rates have risen. The mood of the people is more upbeat. However, we must remain vigilant as the experts tell us that SARS may rear its head again in the winter months. This time around I think we are better prepared and we will not be taken by surprise.

ENG HIN LEE

Dr. Eng Hin Lee is currently Professor in Orthopaedic Surgery and Director, Division of Graduate Medical Studies, National University of Singapore (NUS) and Senior Consultant in the National University Hospital and KK Women's and Children's Hospital. He was previously Head of the Department of Orthopaedic Surgery and Dean of the Faculty of Medicine, NUS. Prof Lee trained in Orthopaedic Surgery in Toronto and specializes in Paediatric Orthopaedics. His research interest is in musculoskeletal tissue engineering and he currently leads the NUS Tissue Engineering Programme. His research has won him the Best Scientific Paper Award from the Paediatric Orthopaedic Society of North America twice in 1993 and 1996, as well as the Yahya Cohen Lectureship in 1999. He is a member of the editorial boards of the *Journal of Paediatric Orthopaedics A & B*, and *Journal of Orthopaedic Surgery and Gait and Posture*. He has over 200 publications in refereed journals.

Section I

WHO: Role and Influence

1

WHO: At the Forefront of Combating SARS

The world's obsession with figures reached a peak in recent months — no thanks to the outbreak of severe acute respiratory syndrome (SARS).

Apart from monitoring share prices, many in the SARS-affected areas have added another item to their daily routine — monitoring the SARS epidemic curve on the WHO website which shows the development of the mysterious disease in various countries.

They check that the number of "active" cases in the hospitals of their countries is below 60; that new SARS cases over a three-day period are kept to fewer than five; that 20 days (or double the longest incubation period) have passed since the last locally acquired case was isolated or died; that there is no community spread of the disease in the country; and that there has not been any exported case. For a SARS-affected area has to meet these requirements to be declared free of the disease by the World Health Organization (WHO). These areas have to prove that their surveillance is reliable too.

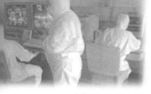

Vietnam was the first country to be announced SARS-free by WHO. It was removed from the organization's list of countries with local transmission of SARS on 28 April.

WHO maintained that the status change for Vietnam was especially significant as it was one of four countries WHO initially identified on March 15 as having local transmission of SARS. Vietnam reported a total of 63 SARS cases and five deaths prior to 8 April.

The Southeast Asian country has proven to have conscientiously implemented detection and protection measures including:

- prompt identification of persons with SARS, their movements and contacts;
- effective isolation of SARS patients in hospitals;
- appropriate protection of medical staff treating these patients;
- comprehensive identification and isolation of suspected SARS cases;
- exit screening of international travelers;
- timely and accurate reporting and sharing of information with other authorities and/or governments.

WHO on Vietnam:
"Since SARS was first detected in Vietnam on 26 February, WHO has collaborated closely with Vietnamese officials to bring the outbreak under control. Key actions have included early recognition of the outbreak, the consolidation of SARS patients in a single hospital, strict infection control, diligent contact tracing, and thorough investigation of all rumoured cases."

Source: WHO website, 28 April 2003

On 12 May, however, WHO began to post on its website a new table indicating those areas with recent local transmission outside a confined setting, such as the healthcare environment. If no new locally acquired cases are identified 20 days after the last reported locally acquired probable case died or was appropriately isolated, the area will be removed from this list. Four patterns of transmission have been identified in this list:

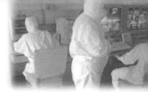

Pattern A

- Imported probable SARS case(s) have produced only one generation of local probable cases, all of whom are direct personal contacts of the imported case(s).

Pattern B

- More than one generation of local probable SARS cases, but only among persons that have been previously identified and followed up as known contacts of probable SARS cases.

Pattern C

- Local probable cases occurring among persons who have not been previously identified as known contacts of probable SARS cases.

Pattern Uncertain

- Insufficient information available to specify the areas or extent of local transmission.

Two recommended measures are specified in the table, which is updated daily: exit screening for international travelers departing the area, and postponing all but essential travel to the area.

Canada's capital Toronto, whose transmission was formerly identified to have followed Pattern B, was removed from the list of areas with recent local transmission on 14 May 2003. Its last locally acquired case was isolated on 20 April.

However, health authorities in Canada informed WHO on 22 May about a cluster of five cases of respiratory illness associated with a single hospital in Toronto. More cases of transmission surfaced. As of 26 June, Toronto continued to experience local transmission of SARS.

The Philippines, which saw 12 probable SARS cases, was next to be removed from the list on 20 May. But another Southeast Asian country, Singapore, was less fortunate. A new SARS case on the 19th day with no infection (which was discovered on 18 May) dashed its hope of following in Vietnam's footsteps. Singapore's health officials notified WHO accordingly and the country's countdown to removal from its list of SARS-affected countries had to start from 11 May, the day the newest SARS patient was hospitalized.

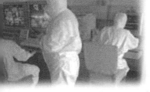

Barely a week before the new SARS case, 30 patients and staff at Singapore's main mental hospital had come down with fever. It was a false alarm then – the patients and staff were diagnosed to have the flu. Undaunted, continued vigilance led the Lion City to be removed from the list of areas with recent local transmission of SARS with effect from 31 May. WHO ceased recommending exit screening of international travelers departing Singapore from that date.

> WHO on Singapore:
> 'From the start, Singapore's handling of its SARS outbreak has been exemplary.... This is an inspiring victory that should make all of us optimistic that SARS can be contained everywhere."
>
> David Heymann, Executive Director
> Communicable Disease, WHO
>
> *Source: WHO website, 30 May 2003*

Besides tracing the development of the disease in SARS-affected areas, WHO issued advisories as early as 15 March, advising that people consider postponing all but essential travel to certain SARS-affected areas.

China, the worst SARS-hit country, was one of the countries which desperately sought affirmation from WHO that it was on the right track towards eradicating the disease. Without such affirmation, countries avoided contacts with it. At one time, more than 100 countries imposed travel restrictions to the mainland.

To help the world's most populous country to battle the infectious disease, a WHO team arrived in China's capital as early as March 23. The investigation team traveled to Guangdong, which was believed to be the first Chinese city to have witnessed SARS (as early as November 2002), in early April. It presented its interim report on the SARS outbreak in Guangdong province on 9 April to the Chinese Minister of Health and Vice-Premier, Wu Yi, in Beijing. It concluded that with "a health system in every hospital at every level", virtually all probable cases of SARS presenting at a hospital in Guangdong province would be detected and rapidly reported.

However, an increase in sporadic cases, which could not be linked to a particular transmission chain, was of particular concern. In Beijing, for example, the authorities indicated inability to trace the origins of many cases. This was especially so as military hospitals are not obliged by Chinese law to report cases to health authorities. Still, a WHO team began visits to Beijing's military hospitals on 16 April. This was followed by an urgent meeting of China's highest ruling body presided over by President Hu Jintao, at which Beijing was explicitly warned against the covering up of SARS cases and instead to ensure "accurate, timely and honest reporting of the SARS situation".

The visits prompted the WHO Beijing team to estimate that the Chinese capital might have as many as 200 cases of SARS, instead of 37 as officially reported. The team recommended that Beijing improve its reporting system, possibly using as a model, procedures followed in Guangdong province, where the daily SARS reports were considered reliable and transparent.

The findings invited much criticism from the international community. The Chinese leadership then decided to view with seriousness, the need for transparency in SARS reporting, and as a consequence, two heads rolled. Beijing's mayor Meng Xuenong, and China's health minister, Zhang Wenkang, were dismissed from key Communist Party posts. Beijing implemented tough measures to contain the disease thereafter, such as imposing quarantines, closing schools and entertainment spots, and even shortening the traditional week-long May Day holiday to a single day. However, records on SARS cases were said to be still flawed.

WHO on Beijing:

"Right now, the situation is that we have a whole load of people (in Beijing) and we don't know where they got the disease…. The problem with the data is that there are holes in it. That means you don't understand what's going on. The epidemic might be flying off in one direction, and you might not know about it."

Mangai Balasegaram
WHO spokeswoman

Source: Associated Press, 10 May 2003

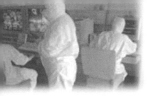

As of 16 May, Beijing has reported less than 50 probable SARS cases for six consecutive days, a far cry from the daily average of more than 100 probable cases from the previous week of April through 3 May. The daily number of new deaths has also declined from a peak of 15 to an average of four.

In mid-May, although the number of new cases in Beijing had dropped from more than 100 in early May to 12 on 19 May, WHO experts cautioned against concluding that the city's SARS cases were on a downward trend. They warned that misdiagnosis of cases could have contributed to the lower number of probable cases. They feared that patients with milder symptoms of SARS or who had no known contact with an infected person were excluded as probable cases.

The number of wrongly diagnosed patients was not known, but WHO experts feared that this could be happening after visits to Beijing hospitals. They were also apprehensive that annual floods in summer might overwhelm the country's sewage system and allow the virus to return with a vengeance. Although the virus did not appear to have spread through water, it could stay in feces for days and that the virus could then be transmitted by overflowing water.

A six-member WHO team of experts was also invited to Shanghai to assess the SARS situation. Among its activities, the team examined the SARS surveillance and reporting system, investigated rumors that the case burden might be higher than officially reported, and visited ten health facilities, three district Centers for Disease Control, and the municipal Center for Disease Control. The team was given free access to all requested data, patient registries, and facilities, which were visited on very short notice.

In its preliminary report of findings in Shanghai, the team found no evidence of systematic underreporting of cases, and concluded that the level of preparedness and response was good. Reporting of cases appeared to be open, frank, and accurate. Over the previous 3–4 weeks, authorities had designated two hospitals as dedicated to the treatment of SARS patients and set up cough and fever clinics. The team also found a very high level of government commitment in tackling the SARS problem.

In addition, a team of four WHO experts took its SARS probe into rural China, where most Chinese live, but where the healthcare system is in a shambles. There were earlier reports that many mainlanders had attacked quarantine sites for fear of the disease.

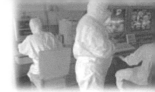

On 9 May, WHO's Director-General, Dr Jong-Wook Lee, arrived in Beijing to exchange views on the SARS situation and other health issues in China. A day before, a WHO team had traveled to Hebei province, which borders Beijing municipality, to assess the SARS situation. WHO had expressed concern that Hebei could be particularly vulnerable to the spread of SARS, as the province has a large population of migrant workers — part of Beijing's "floating population".

As at 15 May, the Chinese provinces of Hebei, Jilin, Hubei, Shaanxi and Jiangsu had been added to the list of affected areas. On the same day, China's Xinhua News Agency quoted Premier Wen Jiabao as saying at a Cabinet meeting, that "no individual or administration will be allowed to tamper with or delay the reporting of information". It added that over 300 Communist Party and government officials had been fired or given other punishments for delaying the release of figures and for other violations in the provinces of Hunan and Jiangsu.

State media also publicized a warning by China's Supreme Court that those who caused death or severe illness by knowingly spreading SARS could face a prison term or possible execution. Quarantine violators could be jailed for up to seven years. A new ruling also stated that information about local emergencies must be passed on from local to provincial to central authorities in just five hours.

WHO's David Heymann traveled to China on 10 June and conferred with health officials about the SARS outbreak and discussed future plans. Both the WHO and the Chinese Health Ministry regarded the emergency response to SARS as an excellent opportunity to strengthen countrywide systems for detecting and responding to all emerging and epidemic-prone infectious diseases. The improvements would strengthen China's capacity to respond to the next influenza pandemic.

WHO on 24 June said it had lifted its travel advisory on Beijing and removed it from the list of areas affected by SARS.

In Hong Kong, as new daily cases continued to fall, local health authorities had since 2 April pursued discussions with the WHO for the territory to be removed from the travel advisory. A mask-burning ceremony should be held to celebrate that, came a suggestion.

On 12 May, in a videoconference with Hong Kong's Secretary of Health, Welfare and Food, Dr Eng-kiong Yeoh, and Director of Health, Dr Margaret

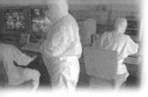

Chan, WHO commended Hong Kong officials for their level of transparency in reporting on the SARS situation in the territory. Hong Kong was taken off the list of SARS-infected areas on 23 June. That certainly called for celebrations, with bars in the popular Lan Kwai Fong district serving free champagne. But the celebrations were largely muted, for the virus had claimed the lives of close to 300 people.

WHO on Hong Kong

"Hong Kong has introduced a rigorous contact tracing procedure. All close contacts of known SARS cases are quarantined at home. In addition, their Hong Kong identity card numbers are passed to the Immigration Department to ensure that these individuals cannot leave the territory."

Source: WHO website, 12 May 2003

Taiwan, on the other hand, was able to quickly trace and isolate the infection sources at the early stages of the epidemic. However, SARS soon spread rapidly within the communities. The number of infected cases accelerated considerably from late April. Not leaving things to chances, Taiwan authorities sealed the Taipei Municipal Ho Ping Hospital after more than 25 suspected SARS cases were discovered, and about 1,100 doctors, nurses, patients and visitors stayed there for up to two weeks. Authorities also sealed off a housing complex where one resident had died of the disease, and one of the largest department stores in Taipei was closed while major a disinfection effort was carried out following the infection of a cashier.

A WHO team arrived on 3 May in Taipei to support the health authorities in combating the SARS outbreak. The two-person team, with expertise in epidemiology and virology, visited hospitals and consulted with local health authorities. On 8 May 2003, WHO issued a warning against nonessential travel to Taiwan's capital.

A day later, when officials could not track down the infection source for a high number of people, WHO upgraded the Taiwanese capital to the category of "high" local transmission of SARS, alongside China's Beijing, Guangdong, Shanxi and Hong Kong.

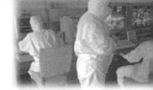

WHO's Dr Heymann said the seriousness of Taiwan's situation lay in the several sources of infection, be they Taiwanese businessmen who had traveled overseas, or healthcare workers who had not had enough knowledge about SARS, among others. To complicate matters, not all organizations and units had joined hands to combat SARS. On 18 May, WHO commented that Taiwan was the territory that had spread the virus most quickly.

Though SARS was an issue concerning public health, Taiwan, which was removed from WHO's list of travel advisory on 17 June, turned it into a viable political weapon. The territory with a longstanding discord with China used the situation to push for some form of representation in WHO.

On 20–21 April, Taiwan hosted a seminar on SARS for the international community. The event was attended by more than 500 health officials and researchers from several countries, and its objective was for information exchange pertaining to the disease. Taiwan's Health Minister, Mr Twu Shiing-jer, used his opening speech for the event to garner support for Taiwan's bid to become an observer in WHO. Taiwan had tenaciously tried to gain WHO observership during the past few years, but its efforts had repeatedly been thwarted by China's objections each year.

In another lobbying effort, Taiwan's representative to the United Kingdom, Mr Tien Hung-mao, argued for Taiwan's participation in WHO in front of the British parliament at a recent international seminar. Mr Tien addressed the House of Commons and expressed Taiwan's aspirations to rejoin WHO, and criticized the "moral unfairness of marginalizing Taiwan from WHO assistance for political reasons".

International indignation against China's earlier mishandling of the SARS outbreak, particularly the cover-up that caused the number of cases to balloon in many countries, turned into greater sympathy for the territory that broke away from the mainland in 1949. The United States, the European Union and Japan all expressed support for an observer status for Taipei at WHO's 56th Assembly held in Geneva from 19 May.

The status was denied, however, following China's strong objection. Only seven friends of Taiwan supported it; those which opposed numbered 27. A week before the meeting commenced in Geneva, both China and Taiwan wrestled for votes. While the former sent Wu Yi to visit WHO's former director-general Dr Brundtland to express gratitude for the organization's repeated visits to various parts of China affected by SARS, the latter had sent

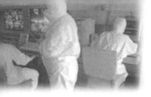

one of its foreign affairs officials on a private visit. During her visit, Wu Yi highlighted the Chinese government's concern for the health of Taiwanese and was active in facilitating interaction between the two places. However, she lamented that Taiwan had politicized the health issue by expressing its willingness to be an observer at the Assembly. Only sovereign states could join WHO, she argued, and Taiwan's effort seemed to be pointing to the creation of a notion of "two Chinas".

Another cross-border meeting which was convened was less controversial. WHO had welcomed the unprecedented efforts made by the Association of Southeast Asian Nations (ASEAN) to coordinate and standardize their campaigns against SARS. Heads of the 10-member association, China and Hong Kong met in Bangkok, Thailand, on 29 April and endorsed a set of procedures to jointly combat the disease. They agreed to standardize the screening of travelers, isolate and treat identified SARS cases, as well as share accurate and timely information.

Addressing participants at the special summit, Dr Heymann reminded the heads of states that there were two simple strategies that could contain and eventually stop SARS — detecting all cases and protecting those at risk of infection from these cases.

"Meetings of this level and magnitude, to formulate a common strategy against a specific disease, show how serious countries are to become free of SARS," he said.

Based on data from Canada, China, Hong Kong, Singapore and Vietnam, WHO had also revised its 6–10% death rate to 15%.

On 26 June, WHO issued a statement to point out that the global public health emergency caused by the sudden appearance and rapid spread of SARS was coming to an end. It expressed optimism that should SARS resurface later this year, the global impact would be milder than experienced during the initial emergency. This is so as the world's public health systems have demonstrated their capacity to move quickly into a phase of high alert, with former SARS hotspots, including Hong Kong and Singapore, planning to maintain a high level of vigilance, supported by measures for screening and detection, until at least the end of the year.

Secondly, the world already has knowledge about what to do. Control measures such as quarantines, though centuries old, have demonstrated their capacity to completely halt the outbreak.

Thirdly, the intensive research effort which is underway, can be expected to improve scientific understanding of SARS and yield better control tools, most notably a rapid and reliable point-of-care diagnostic test.

At the same time, resolutions adopted during the May World Health Assembly allow WHO to move from a passive reliance on official government notifications to a proactive role in warning the world as soon as evidence indicates that an outbreak poses a threat to international public health.

Most important, said WHO, SARS had underscored the importance of immediately and fully disclosing cases of any disease with the potential for international spread. It appears unlikely that any country would choose to conceal cases should SARS resurface. In addition, SARS is simply too big a disease to hide for long.

Section II

China

2

Fighting Infectious Diseases: One Mission, Many Agents

by SHIPING TANG

Combating Infectious Diseases: The Historical Background

Ever since human beings formed communities, infectious diseases have been part and parcel of human experience. For most of our history, we had few effective weapons again these killers, and our species survived largely because of geographical barrier, our immune system, and reproduction capability. Geographical barrier naturally limits the spread of disease, while our immune system gives every individual a chance to survive if he can develop effective immune response to the pathogen in time. Finally, our reproduction capability ensures that our loss of population will be compensated for as time goes by.

After a long period of the existence of tribal communities, mankind embarked on the formation of states, a most powerful institution or organization with an explicit contract between the state and its subjects (people), that the subjects pay taxes in exchange for the state's protection of their lives and property. Protecting people's lives thus became the number

17

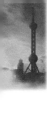
one responsibility of states. Yet, due to lack of effective weapons, states were just as inept as individuals when it came to fight diseases for most of our history.

Not until the invention of the vaccine (against rabies) by Pasteur in 1885 and the discovery of penicillin by Alexander Fleming in 1928, followed by more discoveries of effective antibiotics and vaccines, that we had finally scored a few decisive victories against infectious diseases. But even with the breakthroughs in science and technology in the past century, our capability to win the war against infectious diseases remains limited. Many diseases stay incurable (such as AIDS), while some diseases that were eradicated before have now come back with a vengeance because many pathogens have acquired resistance against previously effective medicines through mutations and natural selection.

The SARS outbreak is just another battle in the ongoing war between human and infectious disease, and it should be understood in the broader historical context outlined above.

States and International Community

One of the factors that contributed to the eventual demise of Athens in its war against Sparta (the Peloponnesian War) in ancient Greece was a severe plaque that wiped out a large population of Athens during a crucial phase of the war.[1] Therefore, although the phrase "non-traditional security" was coined only recently (with SARS clearly fitting into the category),[2] states have long understood that infectious disease is a matter of national security for them. Moreover, as events after the Asian financial crisis and September 11 have indicated, the state remains the most powerful and capable institution in dealing with non-traditional security issues, even if "non-state actors" caused many of the non-traditional security issues. With the advances of science and technology in the past century, states have finally obtained enough tools for combating infectious diseases.

---

[1] For the enduring historical account of the Peloponnesian War, see Thucydides, *The Peloponnesian War*, Rex Warner trans. (London: Penguin Books, 1972).

[2] Mely Caballero-Anthony, "SARS: A matter of national security," *Asia Times*, April 19, 2003.

With our modern day telecommunication and information technology, states can ensure the spread of news about the outbreak of a disease to outpace the spread of the disease itself...

Yet, the advances of science and technology is a double-edged sword for human society. On the one hand, science and technology have brought us vaccines, antibiotics, and more recently, innovative drugs engineered for our war against diseases. On the other hand, science and technology have also brought us steamboat, railway, car, and finally airplanes that greatly diminished the preventive effect of geographical barrier against the spread of disease, and made the restriction of personal movement a far more challenging task than ever before.

The result is that states must now operate under a whole new environment for combating infectious diseases and protecting its subjects' lives, and a new mindset is required.

First, to combat infectious diseases, we need an effective surveillance and early warning system to provide a clear picture of the ground situation, and only a state with its vast network of agents can build such a system. Only with such an effective system can the state hope to draw help from the geographical barrier: With our modern day telecommunication and information technology, states can ensure the spread of news about the outbreak of a disease to outpace the spread of the disease itself so that regions away from the "ground zero" of the outbreak can take preventive measures to prevent or at least slow down the spread of the disease. In contrast, this cannot be easily accomplished in the pre-telecommunication era: more often than not, the spread of the news about an outbreak accompanied the spread of the disease.

Second, to ensure that the dissemination of news of the outbreak outpace the spread of the disease, states must ensure the free flow of this critical information. This should be the critical lesson that China should learn from its experience in this epidemic.

By early February 2003, it became clear that Guangdong had a very serious situation at hand, yet local newspapers in Guangdong were still denying there was a major outbreak of SARS. To make things worse, the Chinese Ministry

In the age of globalization and interdependence, one country's policies often have great consequences beyond its border. China's initial silence on SARS not only jeopardized lives in China, but also those in other infected countries.

of Health did not issue a warning until late March. By then, the epidemic had spread to more than ten provinces (from Guangdong in the south all the way to Beijing and Inner Mongolia in the north), and the situation was already out of control. By maintaining silence on the outbreak and refusing to issue a warning, "China lost the entire month of March in the fight against SARS".[3]

Third, in the age of globalization and interdependence, one country's policies often have great consequences beyond its border (China's initial silence on SARS not only jeopardized lives in China, but also those in other infected countries), and one country's loss does not necessarily translate into other countries' gain. This time, the SARS outbreak not only brought the Chinese economy to a halt, but will also further weaken the strength of world economic recovery in the aftermath of September 11 and the Iraqi war.[4]

Thus, an outbreak of infectious disease is now an international phenomenon with international reverberations, and our effort to contain it must also become international. One country's effort is no longer enough, and the international community must pool their individual resources to win the war.

In particular, because epidemics will remain a geographical phenomenon, affected countries in a particular region especially must work closely with each other and build a regional system for combating infectious diseases. In that sense, ASEAN countries and China must not let the cooperative measures and initiatives against SARS become a one-time ad hoc matter; instead they

---

[3] Henk Bekedam, chief of the World Health Organization (WHO) Beijing office, quoted in Erik Eckholm, "Illness's psychological impact in China exceeds its actual numbers," *New York Times*, April 25, 2003.
[4] Keith Bradsher, "SARS halts expansion of Chinese economy," *International Herald Tribune*, April 28, 2003.

ASEAN countries and China must not let the cooperative measures and initiatives against SARS become a one-time ad hoc matter; instead they should build upon these measures and initiatives and establish a more integrated regional system for dealing with future health crises.

should build upon these measures and initiatives and establish a more integrated regional system for dealing with future health crises.

The 1997 Asian financial crisis propelled the East Asian countries, for the first time in their history, to seriously ponder the vision of an integrated East Asia, and we now have the China–ASEAN free-trade initiative and the "10 + 3" framework. The present SARS epidemic may just drive East Asian countries even closer.[5] If a more transparent government and a free media is SARS's silver lining for China,[6] a more closely linked and cooperative region may be the silver lining for East Asia.

Scientific Community

In the past century, we had witnessed some of the most dramatic advances in science and technology. Yet, science and technology has never been omnipotent or even as potent as people often imagined. For instance, we have long known that the human immunodeficiency virus (HIV) causes AIDS, but after more than ten years of intensive research by the whole scientific community, we still do not have a truly effective treatment for AIDS (the "cocktail" treatment does not cure the disease; it can only control the disease).

---

[5] Thomas Crampton, "Asian leaders map steps to stop SARS," *International Herald Tribune*, April 30, 2003; Marwaan Macan-Markar, "SARS strengthens China–ASEAN ties," *Asia Times*, May 1, 2003.
[6] Shiping Tang, "China looking for SARS' silver lining," *Asia Times*, April 22, 2003.

Unfortunately, the media hype about scientific breakthroughs has created a false sense of security in the general public. Many people now tend to believe that modern medicine engineered from the latest technologies can take care of most of their health problems. The result is that many individuals now live an irresponsible, if not dangerous, lifestyle.

Therefore, other than finding effective cures for more and more diseases, the scientific community has another moral responsibility: to educate the general public and let people know that science cannot solve all the health problems. It must make the public realize that cure always came later than the disease and many diseases killed a lot of people before we could find a cure.

Just like a state cannot always propagate the good news but hold back the bad news, our scientific community also has to report the bad news, rather than just saturating our media with good news. Our scientific community has to acknowledge the limits of science and make the general public aware that certain lifestyles carry inherent dangers to health and science cannot solve all the problems.

In addition, while the scientific community has long established the tradition of international cooperation, international cooperation in scientific community tends to reflect the image of scientists themselves: a lot of personal communication, little institutionalized arrangement.

For purely theoretical, and indeed, for most applied research, the present style of scientific cooperation is not a problem and may even be a plus. For fighting infectious diseases, however, it is no longer adequate.

We need to integrate different national systems of disease surveillance and early warning, disease prevention and scientific research into a global defense system against infectious diseases. This global defense system should be an integrated network of scientific researchers and doctors, backed by states and international bodies. The unprecedented close and speedy cooperation among researchers in nine different countries working on SARS may just have laid the foundation for the future.[7]

Lastly, we need to reform the World Health Organization (WHO) so that it can fulfill its declared objectives under more challenging circumstances (such as the SARS outbreak).

---

[7] Rob Stein, "World's labs unite against viral enemy: Scientists scramble for SARS treatment," *Washington Post*, May 5, 2003.

This global defense system should be an integrated network of scientific researchers and doctors, backed by states and international bodies.

The WHO is part of the larger UN organization, and its decision-making process mirrors that of the UN. WHO's highest decision-making body is the World Health Assembly which is composed of 192 member states: policy implementation is carried out by the Executive Board. The usual decision-making process is that member states submit individual proposals either alone or jointly to the Executive Board. Proposals that receive support from the Executive Board are then presented to the assembly and debated. Unless the assembly can reach a consensus, no decision will be reached no matter how urgent the situation is. While the WHO does have a mechanism for setting up ad hoc open-ended intergovernmental working groups to review the working methods of the Executive Board, there is no office or task force for dealing with emergency issues.

This decision-making process is ill-equipped to deal with emergency issues like Ebola and SARS. At the very least, the WHO needs to set up a task force or office for coordinating all member states' resources in time of emergency. This rapid-reaction task force or group may be best composed of scientists and doctors, and they should be given the authority to determine the degree of urgency of a situation and recommend actions to member states when the Assembly is in recess.[8]

Pharmaceutical Industry

Due to differences in lifesyles, the developed countries tend to have common diseases different from those found in the developing countries (great differences also exist between common diseases in rural and those in urban

---

[8] For similar call for reforming the WHO, see Ilona Kickbusch, "A wake-up call for global health," *International Herald Tribune*, April 29, 2003.

areas in the developing countries). For instance, obesity and cardiovascular diseases are common in the developed countries, while malnutrition and infectious diseases are common in the developing countries, especially in the poor countries in South Asia and the African continent.

Like every business entity, the ultimate measure of success for a pharmaceutical company is its profit. Because the developed countries have more purchasing power and better healthcare systems, it is understandable that most of the giants of the global pharmaceutical industry focus their attention on markets in the developed countries (US, European Union, and Japan), while neglecting those in the developing countries. The result is that diseases in the developing countries received inadequate attention even though the developing countries are home to most of the population on this planet.

Malaria is one such example. Despite that 3000 people die each day in Africa because of malaria, no effective drugs against malaria are reaching there. Unless the international community (especially the developing countries) can work together and force the pharmaceutical industry to face the problem, the situation is unlikely to improve any time soon.

The issue of patent protection for new drugs further complicates the problem. While it is true that patent protection for new drugs is necessary for promoting pioneering research and development of drugs, we are in danger of overdoing it and jeopardizing the ultimate goal of drug discovery in the first place.

Today, global pharmaceutical companies are allowed to charge a premium for a new drug (new chemical entities, or NCEs) under patent protection because they devoted significant resources to research and development for the drug. The result is often that while people in the developing countries are

Because the developed countries have more purchasing power and better healthcare systems, it is understandable that most of the giants of the global pharmaceutical industry focus their attention on markets in the developed countries...

desperate for a new drug, the price charged by global pharmaceutical companies is simply beyond their reach.

To make things worse, global pharmaceutical companies are commercial entities in the developed countries, even though their business interest is already international. They form associations and hire influential lobbies to influence different countries' policies on intellectual property in order to protect their own commercial interests. Without exception, the developed countries backed the pharmaceutical companies' claim that they need a long period of patent protection for a new drug in order to compete, while voices from the developing countries in which people are desperate for medicine are ignored.

However, because the pharmaceutical industry is a global business with implications for the health of us all, regulatory policies on this industry cannot and should not be made by the few developed states in which the pharmaceutical giants are based. Instead, the whole international community must participate in making the rules of this game.

While it is in the short-term interest of the developed countries to grant a long period of patent protection to new drugs, events like September 11 demonstrated that if conditions in the developing countries do not gradually improve, anger and even hatred against the wealthy states would persist and cause major damages. Therefore, it is in the long-term national interest of both the developed and developing countries to reach a compromise between protecting drug patents and saving lives.

At present, there is a mechanism for a state in emergency situations to void still valid patents on drugs and order drugs from companies making the same drugs (called generic drugs).[9] But this does not address the long-term problem of having to pay high prices for drugs that should be more widely distributed. One solution may be for the pharmaceutical companies to make their patents on drugs against infectious diseases more accessible than patents on drugs against non-contagious diseases.

---

[9] For instance, Canadian government ordered generic drugs from Apotex Inc., instead from Bayer A. G., the patent-holder when there was a possible emergency situation of anthrax outbreak in 2001. Amy Harmon and Robert Pear, "Canada overrides patent for cipro to treat anthrax," *New York Times*, October 19, 2001.

25

Individuals

Public health depends on each individual's health in a society, and our individual health will always remain our own problem first. Because drugs cannot solve all of our health problems, our best bet is to do our best to take care of our own health, with medical treatment as our backup.

This means that for our health, we have to re-examine our own behaviors, and see whether some of those behaviors are actually threatening our very own, if not the entire planet's, health.

As it is widely known in China, people in Guangdong seem to have an insatiable and notorious appetite for exotic cuisine made from freshly slaughtered wild animals. This makes the transmission of viruses or other pathogens from animals to humans especially easy.

While the link between animals and human for the present SARS epidemic is not conclusive, at least two threads of evidence suggest that it may be the case: 1) the disease seems to have originated in Guangdong and then spread to Hong Kong (a place with a similar notoriety for exotic diet); 2) patients of the earliest SARS cases reported in Shunde of Guangdong were all working in the catering business. [10]

To minimize future incidents of diseases transmitted from animals to human, the Cantonese people's notorious appetite for exotic cuisine has to have a limit or has to stop. This is not only for the sake of protecting those poor wild animals, but also for the sake of our own health.

On another front, many people's false sense of security about health has translated into more and more people venturing into unexplored territory (the virgin land).

Yet, we know very little about these untainted territories. The caves and jungles must have organisms that we do not know, and if some of them were carried out and brought to the outside world, they could cause diseases against which the general public will have little defense. Ebola virus is one of the primary cases in which a virus normally only associated with primates in African jungle came out to haunt us. HIV is another one.

---

[10] Elisabeth Rosenthal, " From China's provinces, a crafty germ spreads," *New York Times*, April 27, 2003.

People in Guangdong seem to have an insatiable and notorious appetite for exotic cuisine made from freshly slaughtered wild animals.

If we cannot learn the right lesson from the increasingly frequent outbreaks of infectious disease and continue to venture into those territories that we normally do not belong, we are going to pay an even dearer price when one day we came across some other more deadly pathogens.

Today, most of us do not have to explore unchartered territories and hunt for wild beasts as our ancestors had to when facing a growing population and low yield of crops. Most of our adventures into unspoiled territories and hunting for wild animals were for pleasures. While searching for pleasure is our natural instinct, we are not animals. Our search for pleasure must not endanger our own and a whole lot of other species.

Nature is the ultimate master of this planet; we are not. We should show some respect for nature, rather than pretending that we can overrun it. As we have been told again and again, those who do not respect nature will be revenged. SARS is one of a series of warnings that nature has finally struck back.

So it is time for us to cut down some of those irresponsible behaviors and go back to a more humble lifestyle. In some areas, we may need a fundamental change of our behavior.

Lastly, in times of infectious disease outbreaks, each individual's health is no longer a matter of just his or her own concern but a matter of concern for many others. Hence, each individual must do his part for the sake of his own and other's health. Our society cannot tolerate the reckless behavior similar to what an official in Jiangsu province did: he lied to authority and toured four cities after he got back from a trip to Beijing in April, and might have infected as many as 400 people before he was admitted to a hospital. This kind of behavior must be severely punished by law.[11] In fact, if anybody died from contact with him, he should face the charge of manslaughter.

---

[11] Johm Pomfret, "Official's defiance sparks quarantine," *Washington Post*, May 7, 2003.

Wide abuse of medicines means that more and more pathogens will acquire multiple drug resistance, as a recent outbreak of drug-resistant tuberculosis has indicated.

Doctors

Our society has become so dependent on medicine that we are now living in a "drug-ed society", with America as the leading example.

One important reason behind this is that doctors often prescribe medicines even if the patients' own immune system is able to overcome the disease, or prescribe more drugs than the dose needed for curing the disease. Doctors do so because pharmaceutical companies often reward the doctors or hospitals that prescribe their drugs with various kickbacks or perks. This is a common practice in many countries.

This collusion between hospitals, doctors, and pharmaceutical companies means bigger business for the pharmaceutical industry, and we are paying the price, not just financially.

This is because when we take medicines even if our own body can win the battle against pathogens, our immune system will gradually become less robust. Moreover, wide abuse of medicines means that more and more pathogens will acquire multiple drug resistance, as a recent outbreak of drug-resistant tuberculosis has indicated.

The vicious cycle of more drugs leading to less robust immune systems and more drug-resistant pathogens cannot be stopped if doctors continue to prescribe drugs based on incentives rather than necessities.

Additional Reading Recommended

Other than the citations in the footnotes, the general public can find a lot of useful information about infectious diseases on three websites: the World Health Organization (www.who.int), U.S. Center for Disease Control (ww.cdc.gov), and China Center for Disease Control (www.chinacdc.net.cn, for information in Chinese).

SHIPING TANG

Dr. Shiping Tang is Associate Research Fellow and Deputy Director at the Center for Regional Security Studies, Chinese Academy of Social Science, Beijing. He is also co-Director of the Sino-American Security Dialogue.

He has a B.A. in Paleontology from China University of Geosciences (1985), an M.A. in molecular biology from University of Science and Technology of China (1988), a Ph.D. in molecular biology from Wayne State University School of Medicine (1995), and an M.A. in international studies from University of California at Berkeley (1999).

His research falls into two general areas: 1) the psychological dimension of international politics (reputation, credibility, leadership, images, and beliefs); 2) the systematic nature of the security environment and the making of grand strategy. He has published articles in Chinese journals like *China Social Science, Strategy and Management, International Economic Review, World Economics and Politics*, and in English journals like *Asian Survey, Global Economic Review*, and *Journal of East Asian Affairs*. His commentaries have appeared in *Asia Times, China Daily, China Economic Times, Christian Science Monitor, Lianhe Zaobao, Korea Herald*, and *Straits Times*. His book, titled *Grand Strategy: Construct China's Ideal Security Environment*, will be published in 2003–2004.

Contact details:
Dr. Shiping Tang
Deputy Director
Center for Regional Security Studies
Chinese Academy of Social Sciences (CASS)
Beijing
E-mail: twukong@yahoo.com

3

SARS, Anti-Populism, and Elite Lies: Temporary Disorders in China

by *Lynn T. White III**

Rulers in China have for millennia held an odd belief: that natural disasters, such as earthquakes or new diseases, reflect on their legitimacy. Guangdong cadres repressed news of early cases of SARS out of fear that knowledge of this mysterious illness would disturb the populace and sow "disorder" (*luan*). Their delay caused real disorder. Nosy, impolite news reporters might have published data, from the unwashed masses, that would have helped doctors contain the disease early. Elite superstitions about chaos throttled them. More trust of lowlier citizens could have avoided gigantic costs.

* The author thanks the Chiang Ching-kuo Foundation and Princeton University, which provided financial support, and Hong Kong University's Centre of Asian Studies, which provided a desk at which to write. Thanks also go to his sons, Jeremy White and Kevin White, M.D., for their good advice.

The SARS scare raised questions about the efficiency of China's internal structure. These became inseparable from questions about the country's links to the outside world. Xu Zhiyuan, who writes for one of China's economic newsweeklies, claimed that: "SARS has been our country's 9/11. It has forced us to pay attention to the real meaning of globalization.... China's future seemed so dazzling [that it] lulled people into thinking that our country was immune from the shocks of history."[1] Actually, the problem was better blamed on a bug than on history. The virus began in China, and SARS taught at least as much to foreigners as to Chinese about globalization. Unlike the famous flu after World War I, which killed more victims than the war did and was based on a virus that may have developed genetic stability among troops who had been gassed, SARS did not begin internationally.[2] This was a local product, quickly globalized.

All governments face misfortunes that they do not initiate but to which they must react. Beijing has faced other nonpolitical disasters: a 1980 Bohai Gulf drilling rig catastrophe (which was kept secret until the Petroleum Minister resigned), the 1988 hepatitis epidemic in Shanghai, floods in many summers, factory fires, earthquakes, and other calamities. SARS, however, was atypical partly because it hurt intellectuals — especially doctors — and foreign business travelers. Cadres' mistakes and lies were more obviously responsible for its severity.

SARS did not begin with intellectuals, however. One of the first victims was a seller of snakes and birds. He died at the First People's Hospital in Xunde, Guangdong, in December after infecting his wife and several others at that hospital. Other early cases came from the Pearl River Delta cities of Foshan, Xinhui, and Zhongshan, whence a doctor with the virus came to Hong Kong to attend his nephew's wedding.[3] Already in November, odd pneumonias had been reported in Foshan; but some of these were later said to

---

[1] "A New Era in China as SARS Takes Dazzle out of the Future," *International Herald Tribune*, May 14, 2003, New York *Times* report from Erik Eckholm, p. 1.

[2] The WWI flu may have been brought to Europe from an army base in Kansas, apparently gaining virulence in camps and trenches among troops whose respiratory systems had been weakened by gas, then being spread further as troops returned home.

[3] "The Rise of a Virus: From China's Provinces, A Crafty Germ Spreads," report for the New York *Times* by Elisabeth Rosenthal, April 26, 2003, also <http://www.nytimes.com/2003/04/27/health/27sars.html>, May 20, 2003.

be typical rather than SARS.[4] Honest clinical uncertainties were possible in such a situation, even though they could also become a basis for plainly dishonest reporting.

Atypical Medicine versus Typical Economics

The politics of SARS has depended in part on faulty understandings of the genetics of the virus. Many similar bugs, including this one, consist of RNA rather than DNA. Most are "error prone" when they replicate. They mutate quickly; so they can increase or (more usually) decrease in virulence against humans. Even if they become lethal, as the Ebola virus did in Africa, they may kill off their human hosts so quickly that, though highly infectious, they are less often transmitted and can be controlled with quarantines.

Many bureaucrats and political advisors, hoping to minimize embarrassment to themselves as well as govern well, at first thought SARS would be of this type. Some also hoped that the bug's supposed genetic instability might make it a winter season disease (like many flus), so that the onset of summer could aid efforts to eliminate it entirely. Coronaviruses were described as "fragile," and doubts that a mere coronavirus could cause such a persistent disease went together with predictions that such a bug could last only a few hours outside hosts. Statements of this type came mainly from bureaucrats, including those in health ministries, rather than from non-governmental academic epidemiologists, who stressed that little was yet known about the disease.

Policy recommendations that followed this guess that the bug was fragile stressed international advisories against travel. As Toronto's Commissioner of Public Safety said, "The name of this game is that you have to overreact." [5] Early in this process, because some passengers contracted SARS from others sitting near them in airplanes, it was reported that droplets containing the virus might survive even in the extremely dry air of high altitudes and pass through conditioning systems in airplane cabins. Vigorous inbound passenger

---

[4] This information comes from later oral reports, heard in Hong Kong.
[5] Quoted in *SARS War: Combating the Disease*, P.C. Leung and E.E. Oi, eds. (Singapore: World Scientific, 2003), p. 65, and the whole of this pioneering book.

The SARS bug is a typically hardy, in comparison with other viruses of its type.

checks nonetheless began in many kinds of countries only after the virus was already established among local populations. Aviation, tourist, and conference-convention businesses began to hemorrhage huge financial losses. International dealings slowed, in several of the most trade-dependent economies on earth. Businessmen and quality controllers could not visit to make inspections or deals. Tax bases for government revenues plummeted. Land prices continued dropping. Some large and many small firms feared bankruptcy, and a few actually folded. Unemployment rose.

Officials knew that the SARS mortality rate was high (roughly one of every seven reported patients) but not radically higher than in more contagious diseases such as some influenzas.[6] They knew that more people die every two hours from AIDS than (by May 2003) had died in total from SARS, and they knew that the global decimation from malaria was also much worse. They saw that the highly disciplined polity of Vietnam, where the imported case of SARS had been identified early in a single hospital all of whose inmates were strictly quarantined, managed to take itself off the WHO blacklist — so that *if* the Vietnamese border is effectively sealed against future imports of the disease, that country will suffer fewer economic losses. In sum, the view that the bug was genetically unstable led to hopes that severe policies might stamp it out completely, or that it might mutate for the better, fading into history as some previous germs have done.[7]

Medical research by early May showed this hopeful hunch about the genetics of the virus to be wrong: the SARS bug is a typically hardy, in comparison with other viruses of its type. It survives at surprisingly high

---

[6] "Influenza," like "cold," is a broad term, and mortality rates depend on treatment regimes, not just bugs. The comparison above is of current SARS with 1918–1920 influenza. The best available way to calculate the death rate ignores the many subclinical cases and uses data from jurisdictions that do not lie much. Then, over a sizeable sample, take the number of confirmed SARS deaths, and divide by that number plus the number of confirmed SARS discharged/recovered patients. The result is roughly one in seven.

[7] For more, <http://www.newscientist.com/hottopics/sars/article.jsp>, May 20, 2003.

Border defenses and quarantines will help the public if they are maintained.

temperatures (even at 132 degrees Fahrenheit for half an hour), and the onset of summer alone would not reduce it. It can live in feces or other media for days, not hours as had previously been thought. It can create either a gastrointestinal or a respiratory disease. Samples from various countries show, contrary to earlier reports, that there is little or no genetic mutation that might make the germ less lethal; this particular parasite replicates itself all too dependably. Border defenses and quarantines will help the public if they are maintained. This bug can be tamed, but it may prove hard (not impossible) to stamp out totally, especially in poor regions of inland China, until a usable vaccine is developed — and that could take more than a year.[8]

Early policies, based on underestimation of the virus's genetic stability, led to early overconfidence notably in Taiwan, where the Minister of Health on April 10 said that SARS on the island had been "effectively controlled." By May, he had to apologize and resign because the number of SARS cases on his watch, and later, soared. In Singapore, the government managed to reduce the rate of new infections to zero for almost twice the estimated incubation period (as WHO grandees insisted before they would give the city-state a clean bill of health), only to have another case appear at the very end of that time.[9] In Hong Kong, the rate of new infections fluctuated around 60, then 40, then 20, then 30, then 15, and then down and up in single digits for many days. Getting it to zero and keeping it there was difficult, because the bug itself is long-lived and retains its virulence.

---

[8] The genetic stability of the SARS virus makes it less likely to be seasonal, but this is not conclusive because seasonality depends both on the bug and on weather's influence over people's immune systems. SARS's hardiness makes its total elimination more difficult. The future course of this epidemic, like others in the past, could prove to be irregular. An example is the deadly "English sweat" outbreak of the early Renaissance, which disappeared after an extremely uneven and unpredictable career that no epidemiologist has been able to explain; for more on this disease, visit Google.

[9] Because the late Singapore case was a patient who may have caught the bug in Malaysia, WHO did not much delay taking Singapore off its "SARS-affected" list.

> **China has about 400 million smokers whose lungs have been weakened by this habit, in part because state agencies are addicted to revenues from cigarette sales.**

These relatively rich polities will almost surely succeed in controlling SARS, as Chinese cities will, but eliminating the virus from the whole planet is less certain. China's rural health system is weak. Some analysts opine that China's spending for health (if the reported budgets are accurate) is less than the PRC's other indices of modernization would predict. Diseases such as tuberculosis, AIDS, neonatal tetanus, lead poisoning, and hepatitis B are high, for a low-medium income country.[10] Tobacco addiction is widespread. China has about 400 million smokers whose lungs have been weakened by this habit, in part because state agencies are addicted to revenues from cigarette sales. Compared with most of Africa, the rural health system in China (as in almost every other country) looks good. The rural PRC is, however, better prepared to distort reports about this disease than to eliminate it wholly. Policies based on hopes that the germ might be unstable were not wrong, despite later information that it is all too stable. These policies will be continued. The notion that the epidemic might be stopped with a quick slap, however, was misconceived. SARS must be treated together with other long-term issues.

The main problem was the economic effect of media overreaction to the very human story of SARS deaths. David Baltimore, a virologist who won a Nobel prize in medicine and is president of Caltech, railed against media for alarmism about SARS, as distinct from other hazards, in countries where its incidence was relatively low. As he said, "The media believe — and I can't say they're wrong — that people just enjoy being scared. And because their readers and viewers enjoy it, the media play to it."[11]

---

[10] China's AIDS rate, as part of its very large population, is uncertain; reporting is incomplete. Data on overall medical delivery are also hard to confirm; but improvements in medicine have clearly not kept up with economic improvements in recent decades.

[11] "Regarding Media: A Plea for Careful SARS Coverage," Los Angeles *Times*, April 30, 2003, p. 1.

The economic costs of this particular sort of overreaction have been gigantic. SARS has produced its quota of gallows humor; some wags say the acronym really stands for "Severely Affected Retail Sales." The Asian Development Bank made a preliminary estimate that SARS could cost Asia $28 billion: 4 percent of total GDP in Hong Kong, approximately 2 percent in Taiwan and Singapore, about 0.5 percent in China (where the service sector, hardest hit by SARS, is relatively less important than manufacturing).[12] Some argue that the nasty bug could also cause nasty, anti-Asian, autarkic economics in the United States. The SARS recession could reduce demand in Asia for American goods more than it decreases exports from Asia to America. By mid-2003, the U.S. trade deficit was running at $500 billion per year, a rate that is unsustainable for very long. Most of the deficit is with East Asia, not with Europe or NAFTA. It is mostly caused by U.S. imports of manufactures that partially displace goods produced by American workers. Because the Chinese RMB and the Hong Kong dollar are pegged by those governments to the greenback, and because upward valuation of the Taiwan dollar has also been limited by official actions, "Asian nations are laying themselves open to retaliation through arbitrary [U.S.] measures that would be more damaging to their global trade prospects. They may be creating conditions for 1930s-style competitive devaluations and the resurgence of protectionism."[13]

In Hong Kong, the large middle-income stratum of people with white collar jobs, serving companies whose blue collar workers are mostly in Guangdong, were economically frustrated even before SARS appeared. Many such families have negative equity in their main assets, their flats. People in this group owe more to banks than the value of the collateral on which they took out mortgages. SARS makes their indebtedness worse, even if they can keep their jobs, because it further depresses the value of their flats. They are scared of the bug (although few catch it), and they are furious at their loss of wealth. They tend to blame the local Government, which does not have the strength to make big allocative decisions that a provable popular mandate might give them. Top officials, promising wisdom and effectiveness even though nobody

---

[12] "SARS Could Cost Asia $28bn.," BBC News, May 9, 2003, 9:05 GMT.
[13] See Philip Bowring, "How SARS could Cause a Trade War," *International Herald Tribune*, May 15, 2003, p. 6.

could perform perfectly under such circumstances, tend to undermine their own credibility.

It is not a defense of the self-interested and overly proud tycoons who run most of East Asia to point out that economic depression can mean human tragedy no less surely than medical plague can. Public fright of SARS, together with a tendency by media to make sales from scary news, meant that the real dangers of SARS were not considered together with endemic medical dangers — or together with economic dangers arising from gestures that were medically ineffective but politically gratifying. If governments had understood earlier not just that the virus is persistent, but also that public campaigns against it needed to be calm and focused enough for sustainability, these costs might have been somewhat lessened.

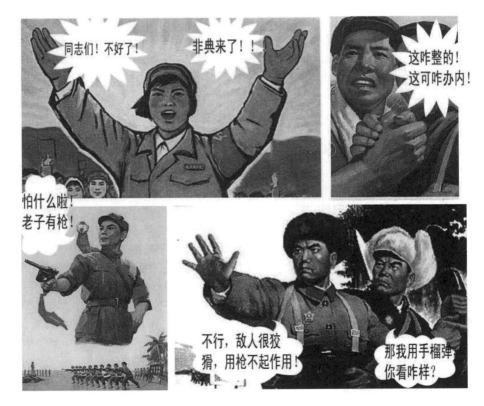

Public fright: villagers first thought SARS can be eradicated by gun and grenade.

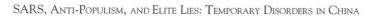

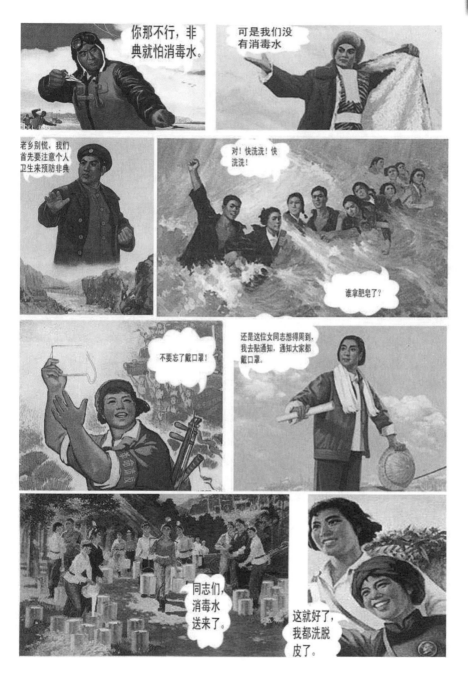

Personal hygiene as the key to fighting SARS: the use of disinfectant, masks, etc.

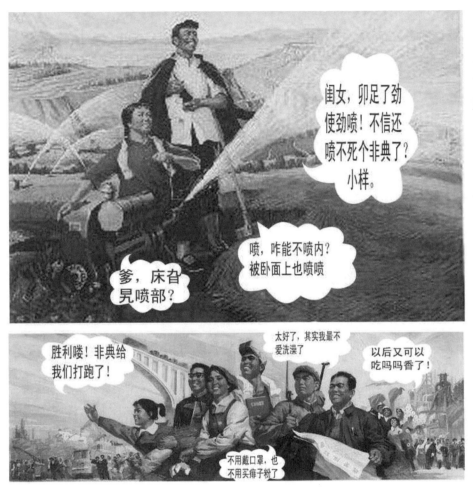

Villagers rejoice because of victory over SARS.

The bug was, however, the political problem of the day. Other hazards, including some that are equally fatal and some that leave people unemployed or poor (and thus more vulnerable to further distresses, including other diseases), were less novel. So they were less often brought to public attention and were not considered together with SARS. Elites were so interested in using SARS to prove the general truths of either liberal or illiberal forms of government, they performed rituals to those ends more than they sought any focused long-term cures. Bureaucrats were so hopeful of swatting the virus, they failed to cue citizens to the whole panoply of social opportunities and problems. They were schizophrenic about the medical and the economic costs, finding it easier to attempt statistical lies about the epidemic than to find a coherent set of medical-cum-economic policies that could be sustained over a long time. They needed to persuade large numbers of people to help quarantine the bug, without incurring any unnecessary economic losses.

Factional Analysis versus Social Analysis

SARS came in a guise to challenge the centrist structure of the Chinese state. It began in the second-farthest province from the capital. It was an upwelling of "chaos" such as most directly defies the image of China as, in principle, homogeneous and small, like a point (Beijing) rather than a plane with many parts. All broadly social fields, including economic development, are of course regionalized to a great extent. China's politics is not so widely spread, however, in the minds of most who write about it.

In a prominent *Newsweek* magazine article, Harvard professor Roderick Macfarquhar depicted "the image of China's leaders behaving in feckless fashion, putting politics before people. The leadership's perennial obsession with secrecy led it to prevaricate about the extent of the disease in the capital for five months." Questions about who knew what, how clearly, and when are frequent in investigations of bad leadership. (Senior readers will recall these from the Watergate era.) Was *anybody* in Beijing aware of the existence of this disease during the Sixteenth Party Congress in November 2002? Evidence to answer that question is unavailable in public, and probably in private too. Could the bugs have paid so little attention to such important politics?

Could the bugs have paid so little attention to such important politics?

41

Macfarquhar wrote that,

> The public-health crisis is beginning to pull back the curtain that hides the divisions within the party itself. Clearly, the honeymoon is over for the new leaders, President Hu Jintao and Premier Wen Jiabao. Whether praise for the energetic measures they have taken to contain the epidemic outweighs blame for concealing it will doubtless depend on the human toll SARS extracts.... But for China's leaders, the popular mood will be of less consequence than the factional struggle within the party.[14]

The People's Republic is no democracy, to be sure. Evidence thus far fails to show, however, that SARS will throw into fierce struggle the latent factions that exist in its top leadership (as in all governments). Is a *coup d'état* expected?[15] Many recent writers, not just Macfarquhar, have used logical frameworks that are based not on contemporary data, but on extrapolations to 2003 of notions about the structure of China's top politics for which the most recent sure evidence is more than a dozen years old, and most of the evidence is over a quarter century old. Scholars who have experience in governments know how sharp bureaucratic disputes can become. They could, however, put this accurate understanding into more social and long-term perspective.

Has China changed at the top? Practically all of its networks have changed a great deal in the past decade and more. Is the leadership an exception? Even the top leaders may well be unsure. If we want to focus on that "level" of

---

[14] Roderick Macfarquhar, "Unhealthy Politics," *Newsweek*, May 12, 2003, p. 18.

[15] Some Asian countries have had many coups. Using logic such as is criticized above, it would have been simple to show, for example, that Thailand could not possibly have passed its financial crisis without a coup. Thai soldiers had often toppled governments with far less excuse. Yet Bangkok saw no coup in 1997. As a future book by this author will show, more widespread structural changes of leadership (in that case, a rise of Sino-Thai provincial politicians who could command electoral majorities) had by then altered the basic form of that country's top politics. For discussion of such a tectonic shift in the late great USSR, see Seweryn Bialer, *Stalin's Successors* (Cambridge: Cambridge University Press, 1980). For a parallel argument about contemporary China, see the next footnoted source, which relies mainly on statistical analysis of the traits of many leaders, not just two or three or seven.

Guangdong Party Secretary Zhang Dejiang — suppressed *both* public and governmental reporting of the epidemic until it could no longer be hidden.

politics (ignoring Speaker Tip O'Neill's greater wisdom that "All politics is local"), the most obvious fact about these men is that they are technocrats. Every last member of the Politburo Standing Committee is an engineer. None are soldiers.[16] Hu Jintao is no Mao Zedong. Dull Jiang had as much charisma as Hu, and he was promoted to power when Deng Xiaoping led the country.

Perhaps Macfarquhar and most other expert analysts are correct to posit "endemic factionalism in the leadership... driven more by personality than policy.... The SARS epidemic could be the catalyst for the struggle to begin now [early May 2003]." Perhaps "the military's insubordination in the early stages of the crisis may be an opportunity for Hu to whittle away Jiang's power base."[17] Very many Chinese intellectuals in the PRC, Hong Kong, and elsewhere take a similar line. They underestimate, too hopefully from the viewpoint of the social status of intellectuals, the degree to which their country has changed. In any case, evidence that SARS should be deemed mainly about factional struggle, rather than about regime legitimacy and policies to control a nasty virus, is thus far weak. If factional conflict were to break out, it is incidentally also unclear what side might deserve support. The Chinese government no doubt still needs moral harangues from intellectuals, but these could be more useful if they concerned actual problems.

Evidence suggests that top Beijing politicos did not hear about SARS as a serious disease until February 2003, and that provincial cadres — notably Guangdong Party Secretary Zhang Dejiang — suppressed *both* public and governmental reporting of the epidemic until it could no longer be hidden. On the very first day of the year, a Guangdong provincial health team was sent to the city of Heyuan, 100 miles northeast of Guangzhou, where five people

---

[16] See Li Cheng and Lynn White, "The Sixteenth Central Committee of the Chinese Communist Party: Hu Gets What?" *Asian Survey* 43: 4 (July/August 2003), lead article.
[17] Macfarquhar, "Unhealthy Politics," p. 19.

had been infected by a shrimp salesman who had later passed the virus to others in Guangzhou. On January 27, the Guangdong health department received a "top secret" report, apparently from this team, about the new pneumonia. Nobody yet knew its pathogen.[18]

At the end of January, the province medical department informed Guangdong hospitals of the outbreak, but "authorities did not want concerns about the virus to cut into people's spending during the Chinese New Year holiday." [19] When did anybody official in Beijing hear? The *Southern Daily* later claimed that Guangdong did not report the outbreak to the central government until February 7. Two days later, a team headed by Deputy Health Minister Ma Xiaowei was sent south. Many in Guangdong cities who had internet connections or mobile telephones learned about SARS between February 8 and 10. Provincial Party Secretary Zhang tried to suppress the news that the *Guangzhou Daily* and other media nonetheless publicized on February 11.

A Shanxi jewellery dealer, who caught SARS in Guangdong during February, returned home to her provincial capital, Taiyuan. She infected several people there (including her parents, who both died); but she was dissatisfied with the quality of her treatment in that relatively poor province. This "superspreader" had enough clout or money to move to Beijing's No. 301 Military Hospital, infecting yet more people.

On March 9, after the opening of the National People's Congress, the Ministry of Health explicitly ordered the heads of Beijing hospitals to report SARS cases only through channels upward on a confidential basis, but *not* to any media. At the NPC itself, however, thirty Guangdong delegates "offered a motion to establish a nationwide epidemic prevention network, a circuitous signal of their concern." When a Guangzhou paper published a March 6 article saying the virus was not under control, local Party chief Zhang "forced the paper to pull its reporter from Beijing and threatened to shut the paper down, media sources said." [20] On March 15, the CCP Propaganda Department ordered

---

[18] "China's Slow Reaction to Fast-Moving Illness," Washington *Post* Foreign Service report by John Pomfret, April 3, 2003, p. A18.

[19] "Outbreak Gave China's Hu an Opening: President's Move on SARS Followed Immense Pressure at Home, Abroad," Washington *Post* Foreign Service report by John Pomfret, May 13, 2003, p. A01.

[20] "Outbreak Gave China's Hu an Opening," loc. cit.

Speaking truth to power is a virtue that can easily be described in terms of " Chinese characteristics," just as the equally ancient tradition of bureaucratic lying can.

newspapers not to report the WHO's first global warning about SARS. E-mails and text messages spread this international report widely, even though China's newspapers could not publish it.

The severity of the outbreak in Beijing was probably related to the salience of military hospitals there, to the frequent migrations of people from nearby Shanxi and Hebei, and to the timing of the pre-scheduled NPC just as a wave of infections arrived in the capital. On April 2, WHO advised against travel to Hong Kong or Guangdong. On the next day, Health Minister Zhang Wenkang said in a news conference that China was "safe" and that Beijing had just twelve SARS cases. But on April 4, a 72-year-old retired doctor and Party member from the Beijing No. 301 Military Hospital named Jiang Yanyong, sent e-mails to the Central TV network in Beijing and to Phoenix TV in Hong Kong, reporting at least 100 cases in Beijing. Neither station publicized this report, but someone leaked it to *Time* magazine, which put these data on a website by April 9. The fact of the Health Minister's lie was thus sent back, throughout China.

Dr. Jiang was brave enough to protest the cover-up of SARS and challenge official falsehoods. He later opined that, "In China, we have said too many lies for too long. All I did was tell the truth. I did nothing special."[21] This modesty was in the style of loyal Confucian *literatus*, as was his original remonstrance. Speaking truth to power is a virtue that can easily be described in terms of "Chinese characteristics," just as the equally ancient tradition of bureaucratic lying can. The PRC government has usually stressed China's "uniqueness" as "a construct that is manufactured to fend off any critical efforts to measure China against anything that is called democratic," as Anita Chan

---

[21] Allen T. Cheng, "Doctor who Exposed Cover-Up Wins Official Recognition," *South China Morning Post*, May 17, 2003, p. A3 — but when that reporter attempted a follow-up interview with Dr. Jiang, Party officials at his military hospital refused to give permission.

Chinese intellectuals jump to factional interpretations of *everything* social. This phenomenon also calls for explanation.

notes.[22] But ambiguous uniqueness is just another official fib. Asian values come in many forms.

On April 17, Hu Jintao called a meeting of the Politburo (the Party's 25 highest-ranked officials). According to one report, he "acknowledged that the government had lied about the disease."[23] Hu and Wen Jiabao clearly gained more distinct profiles for themselves among many Chinese, as they worked publicly in the spring of 2003 against SARS. On April 20, the government admitted serious past mistakes in reacting to the disease. The Mayor of Beijing and the Minister of Health were credibly senior scapegoats, sacked because they had caused damages by hiding information. Many others at lower ranks and in Guangdong were surely at least as remiss. A few of these also lost their jobs. But the bugs, showing serious *lèse-majesté*, continued to spread.

Shortly after the order for transparency went out, 26 of China's 31 provinces reported SARS cases, although the completeness of these reports was subject to many doubts. There was more political than epidemiological discourse on the distinguished dismissals. The deposed Minister of Health Zhang Wenkang had long associations with Jiang Zemin, but the deposed Mayor of Beijing Meng Xuenong, with Hu Jintao. So there seemed to be equal opportunity, among the apparent factions, in these sackings. This may be complex, however, because Meng had become unpopular in some quarters for his earlier policies toward "Zhejiang village" in Beijing. The capital is of such importance in the Chinese polity that the severity of SARS there, on his watch, was an embarrassment even though his administration could not control military hospitals. Still, many believe that Meng should not have been dismissed. A Beijing newspaper editor was reported to have said anonymously: "Yes, Beijing did underreport its SARS figures, but who else did not? Why were there not

---

[22] Anita Chan, "The Changing Ruling Elite and Political Opposition in China," in *Political Oppositions in Industrializing Asia*, Garry Rodan, ed. (London: Routledge, 1996), p. 161.

[23] "Outbreak Gave China's Hu an Opening, loc. cit.

sackings in Guangdong, Hunan, or Shanghai?"[24] These were good questions, even though Chinese intellectuals jump to factional interpretations of *everything* social. This phenomenon also calls for explanation, but it does not prove in any particular case whether they are right or wrong. Evidence is always needed, for that.

Premier Wen Jiabao was more closely connected with his predecessor Zhu Rongji than with either the Hu or Jiang group. Factional analysis works best with just two sects (because, in principle, factions conflict on all issues and need maximal support to win). Perhaps nobody whosoever knows exactly how many there may be, currently, at the "top" in Beijing.

Xinhua News Agency announced on April 24 that a State Council meeting had established the SARS Control and Prevention Headquarters, chaired by "Iron Lady" Vice-Premier Wu Yi, to stamp out the disease and upgrade county level hospitals. Jiangsu Province by May 4 deployed 17,000 police to check the temperatures of everyone entering the province by air, sea, or land. Police teams were sent to any village where fevers were reported.[25] Other provinces acted similarly.

By May 7, the Ministry of Health issued "special regulations designed to strengthen the monitoring of workers returning to the countryside from SARS epidemic areas," which at that point included Guangdong, Beijing, Shanxi, Inner Mongolia, and Hebei.[26] Migration controls may, because illegal migrants hide, actually make SARS control more difficult. This has been the case even on Taiwan, which is cut off from the mainland by 160 kilometers of water and political separation. A SARS hotspot, nonetheless, is the relatively poor district of Wanhua, Taipei, which includes old buildings and "many illegal immigrants who can evade the quarantine nets: they do not enter Taiwan by going past the airport's thermal camera, but hidden aboard fishing boats."[27]

Some Chinese intellectuals hoped that the epidemic might improve their country's governance. Trying to rescind the official tradition that information about disasters should be kept secret, Premier Wen Jiabao in mid-May, 2003,

---

[24] See <http://www.atimes.com/atimes/china/ed24ad01.html> for Xu Yufang, "China's Atypical Politics," accessed on May 20, 2003.

[25] See <http://www.news.sina.com.cn/c/2003-05-04/23581030013.shtml>, May 20, 2003.

[26] Personal communication from an informant whom this author thanks.

[27] "Taiwanese Chafe at SARS Quarantine," *International Herald Tribune*, May 13, 2003, New York *Times* report of Donald G. McNeil, Jr., p. 4.

signed a regulation that, "The release of information must be swift, accurate, and comprehensive."[28] Reports on epidemics were henceforth to be sent immediately to high levels in Beijing. More important, officials and newspapers were ordered to provide the public with such news. Officials evading these rules were threatened not just with dismissal, but also with criminal charges.

It was far less certain whether such rules could be enforced, and whether these regulations extended to news other than epidemic infections. Vice-Minister of Health Gao Qiang on May 30 damned Dr. Jiang Yanyong with faint praise for having blown the whistle on earlier lies: "we have six million health care workers.... Jiang is just one of them." Opposition to his view, however, made Jiang a public hero; by mid-June, his face was on the front of a popular newsweekly over the caption, "Jiang Yanyong: The interests of the people are more important than anything."[29] Some Westerners called on Chinese leaders to follow Gorbachev's explicit realization, after Chernobyl, that the disaster showed the Communist system to be broken.[30] The CCP leaders were very unlikely to take such advice, in light of what followed for Gorbachev.

China's slightly greater transparency in 2003 has not been strictly limited to SARS, although its extent can easily be overstated. After seventy sailors on a training course in Submarine 361 suffocated (apparently because the diesel engine, using oxygen, was not shut down during a dive), this news was made public. Disasters, especially military ones, had practically never before been reported in China. So the announcement of this tragedy, which did not include its date, broke a tradition. The families of the deceased sailors, if ordered to maintain military silence, would probably have remained quiet. By May 5, 2003, the sub was towed to its base near Dalian. Jiang and Hu, who are often described as the top leaders of China's main conflicting factions, were shown together on TV, touring the refloated sub and consoling relatives of the deceased together.[31]

---

[28] "Beijing Issues Strict Rules on Reporting Epidemics," *International Herald Tribune*, New York *Times* report from Erik Eckholm, May 14, 2003, p. 1.

[29] "China to Open Field in Local Elections: Decision to Allow Multiple Candidates Comes During Debate Over Need for Reform," by John Pomfret, Washington *Post* Foreign Service, June 13, 2003, p. A18.

[30] This was the thrust of an editorial in the *International Herald Tribune* on May 21, 2003. p. 8.

[31] "China's Leaders' Grief on Display: Submarine Disaster Brings New Move Toward Official Candor," *International Herald Tribune*, May 7, 2003, from a New York *Times* report by Erik Eckholm and an Agence France Press report, p. 8.

There is extensive evidence of cooperation among high Chinese leaders who can be assigned to different factions. Hu Jintao and Zeng Qinghong (who is widely seen as Jiang Zemin's younger stalking horse) are the past and current presidents of the Central Party School, where their cooperation has been frequent and so publicized that some will doubt its sincerity on that ground. They have handed out degrees to graduates together. They have made speeches in praise of each other's ideas.[32] As far as scholars can know now, at least, they conflict less than Colin Powell and Donald Rumsfeld do, for example.

In late spring, there was still extensive evidence that mid-level Chinese officials in many provinces were suppressing news. There were so many of these cadres, as reported by callers to Western media in China, not all could conceivably have been known to any top leader.[33] There are more certain signs of conservative inertia in the huge Chinese bureaucracy than of vicious power struggle among its top leaders, even though both Chinese and Western writer-intellectuals pay more attention to the potential factionalism.

The question is not whether latent leadership divisions exist in China. They exist in all governments. The question, instead, is whether Beijing's factions still forebode as much elite violence as was evident in the late 1960s or perhaps the somewhat less extreme house arrests and jailings of 1989.[34] There is a halting and slow historical trend for the better on this score, and it relates to much wider sociopolitical change in China.

"Mr. Science" versus "Mr. Democracy"

Broad-based social transformation has been occurring in this country for many decades, on roughly the same course since the early 1970s at least.[35] This

---

[32] For much more, see Li and White, "The Sixteenth Central Committee," loc. cit.

[33] "Telling the Truth about SARS from Inside China," *Asian Wall Street Journal* commentary by Jennifer Chou, May 9, 2003.

[34] The bloody violence of 1989, in which more ordinary citizens than young intellectuals died, can be put in perspective of the data about high elites in Michael Schoenhals, "The Organization and Operation of the Central Case Examination Group (1966–1979): Mao's Mode of Cruelty," *China Quarterly* 145 (March 1996), pp. 87–111.

[35] See Lynn White, *Unstately Power: Local Causes of China's Economic Reforms* (Armonk: M.E. Sharpe, 1998).

Similar elites overspecify the truth, using it to persuade themselves they must keep others from power.

change has too seldom been recognized, because talk of its political effect is officially taboo. It has negative implications for the social status of intellectuals as distinct from entrepreneurs, of residents in Beijing and other provincial capitals as distinct from people who live elsewhere, and of cadres as distinct from citizens. As Ronald Inglehart writes, "Since coercion and culture are simply different aspects of political power, the elite most dominant in any society (after the military) is the priesthood or the other ideologues who provide the authoritative interpretation of the society's cultural norms."[36] In China, this elite has for centuries been the intellectuals. "The enlightened awake the others," according to Mencius. Accredited, educated people credibly form a natural elite. In China, they have followed traditions inherited from their predecessors both in traditional Confucian times and in the anti-traditional May 4 Movement that glorified "Mr. Science" (Cai xiansheng) and "Mr. Democracy" (De xiansheng). They have studiously ignored the anti-democratic aspects of the notion that credentialed knowledge confers a right to rule.

Various kinds of learning have been seen at different times to legitimate government: knowledge of Confucian ethics, as tested by "eight legged" essays, was prerequisite for powerful posts in the civilian bureaucracy in many imperial eras.[37] Knowledge of modern styles and "scientism" was important for civilian posts in the time of the republic. In all periods, militarists had power too.[38] In current China, knowledge of engineering is deemed so legitimate that every member of the country's highest decision-making body, the Politburo Standing

---

[36] Ronald Inglehart, *Modernizations and Post-Modernizations: Culture, Economics, and Politics in 43 Countries* (Princeton: Princeton University Press, 1997), p. 55.
[37] Confucian knowledge came in both adaptive and brittle forms, which are beautifully described by Joseph Levenson, *Confucian China and its Modern Fate: The Problem of Monarchical Decay* (Berkeley: University of California Press, 1964).
[38] See Danny W.Y. Kwok, *Scientism in Chinese Thought, 1900–1950* (New Haven: Yale University Press, 1965).

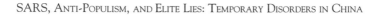

Committee, has an engineering degree.[39] Similar elites overspecify the truth, using it to persuade themselves they must keep others from power.

When the early socialist Chen Duxiu introduced "Mr. Democracy" and "Mr. Science," he declared that, "We are now quite sure that only these two gentlemen can save China and get rid of all political, moral, academic, and ideological darkness." [40] Chen called for a "new ideology." Its elements were to be "science" and "human rights" (he later changed the political element to "democracy"). Chen argued that, "After the rise of science, its role will not be less than that of the theory of human rights," and he posited that the two would be "a chariot with two tires." But democracy, as his waffling about it suggests, was harder for him to conceive than science.

Chen downplayed the extent to which traditional China had developed science.[41] He stressed that peasants should choose good seeds and fight insects; workers also needed science to avoid wasting materials so that China would no longer have to depend on foreign war material; and businessmen needed it so they would not seek short-term interests and could calculate better for the future.[42] The aim of such science was not truth, but national strength — for a state that should still be run by an intellectual elite.

Student banners at Tiananmen in 1989 on the anniversary of May 4 lamented, "Seventy years already!" and "We have waited too long for Mr. Science and Mr. Democracy!" [43] By stressing "Mr. Science" rather than deconstructing the interests of a scientific elite, Chinese intellectuals have obscured the connection between imperial norms and their own new social situation. By criticizing Confucian traditions selectively, they have likewise neglected the democratic potential in Mencius's doctrine of a "natural mandate"

---

[39] See Li and White, "The Sixteenth Central Committee," Table 2. No member of the Standing Committee is military; most of the non-military members of the whole Politburo were also educated as engineers.

[40] Chen Duxiu, "Xin qingnian zuian dabian" ("Defense of the New Youth Case"), *Xin qingnian* (New Youth) vol. 6, no. 2., in *Chen Duxiu wenzhang xuanbian* (Selected Works of Chen Duxiu) (Beijing: Sanlian Shudian, 1984).

[41] Joseph Needham, *Science and Civilization in China* (Cambridge: Cambridge University Press, various years).

[42] *Xin qingnian* (New Youth), September 15, 1915.

[43] Vera Schwarcz, "Memory, Commemoration, and the Plight of China's Intellectuals," *Wilson Quarterly* (Autumn 1989), p. 121.

(*tianming*). As a Western democrat has written, "Of course, Mencius... emphasized patriarchal virtues such as filial piety and the subordination of women. Yet his radical belief in the goodness of human nature and in the 'right of rebellion' has inspired popular uprisings and frightened aristocrats from his day forward." [44]

Some of China's most prominent intellectuals who think they are democrats are in fact not so. Philosopher Li Zehou argued in 1989 that "democracy must be more scientific." [45] The famous astrophysicist dissident Fang Lizhi once said, "Because science and technology have become more and more important in the world in which we are living, there are a great many problems that only people with some background in science or culture may be able to grasp clearly." [46] This is true, but it is not enough to establish a structure in which science will serve most people. Modernistic journals in China's most liberal recent period during the late 1980s, such as the *World Economic Herald,* clearly plumped for rule by intellectuals.[47] That newspaper (banned in 1989) discussed "China's Modernization and the Ideological Trend of Populism," arguing *against* the populist trend.[48] Most Chinese educated people like to claim that "the masses" caused violence during the Cultural Revolution. They have unpresentable social reasons to forget that young ambitious intellectuals were at the very forefront in that disaster of the late 1960s.

Democracy arises when leaders change: when they become less interested in publicizing the lie that they understand a permanent cosmic morality. They become less naïve in suggesting that they have a single key to all knowledge, when they become more needful of compromises among themselves as leaders of various different, larger social groups. A student of the messy American

---

[44] Roger V. Des Forges, "Democracy in Chinese History," in Des Forges, Luo Ning, and Wu Yen-bo, eds., *China: The Crisis of 1989* (Buffalo: State University of New York, 1990), pp. 29–30.

[45] "*Minzhu yao kexue hua,*" Vera Schwarcz, "Memory," p. 124.

[46] Christopher Buckley, "Science as Politics and Politics as Science: Fang Lizhi and Chinese Intellectuals' Uncertain Road to Dissent," *The Australian Journal of Chinese Affairs* 25 (January 1991), p. 16.

[47] See Li Cheng and Lynn White, "China's Technocratic Movement and the *World Economic Herald,*" *Modern China* 17: 3 (July 1991), 342–388.

[48] *Shijie jingji daobao,* May 1, 1989, p. 1.

" Mr. Science" betrays his former friend, " Mr. Democracy."

polity has written, "Democracy is a political system for people who are not sure that they are right." If leaders are always presumed to preach comprehensive truths — as most Chinese intellectuals like to suggest, although most ordinary Chinese know better — this impedes their candidness to admit that, over many issues and in the long term, "nobody knows enough to run the government." [49]

Chinese educated people — governmentalists and dissidents alike — nonetheless continue to opine that for China to be strong, the nation must be run by a knowledge elite (*zhishi jingying*). This notion puts off competitive elections that might also empower entrepreneur, labor, and farmer leaders. It encourages "movement democracy," whose sporadic outbursts have no lasting effect on decision-making structures. Cultural, economic, educational, and demographic conditions in China would certainly, already or within a couple of decades at least, sustain more liberal structures. But they will not do so until the usual scenario of liberal transformation begins. An urban populace, supported by some military and police, shields a group of intellectuals who decide operate a constitutional framework providing popular choice between competitive elites. The result would be leaders who may be educated but are not intellectuals before all else. Until then, "Mr. Science" betrays his former friend, "Mr. Democracy."

If China attains 5 percent real growth for two more decades, it will have a level of per capita wealth above which no democracy has ever been overthrown. [50] Especially because China is a very large and ethnically unchallenged country (different from Singapore, for example), an elite decision to liberalize well before that time, even now, would almost surely be permanent — and it *might* be taken, if most Chinese intellectuals were not so

---

[49] E.E. Schattschneider, *The Semi-Sovereign People: A Realist's View of Democracy in America* (Hinsdale, IL: Dreyden Press, 1960), intro. by David Adamany, pp. 54–133.
[50] Adam Przeworski *et al.*, *Democracy and Development, 1950–1990* (Cambridge: Cambridge University Press, 2000), p. 273.

> **Toronto, Singapore, the Philippines, New York City, Vietnam, Taiwan, and Beijing clearly show that success against SARS depended on the timing of quarantines, not on the elites' preferred political philosophies.**

disdainful of most of their compatriots. Non-elites cannot create democracy without support from elites, and in China that definitely means educated people.[51]

A shift to democracy is precisely the kind of decision that most Beijing intellectuals resist because of their self-serving antipopulism. They deem "the masses" unfit for politics. They live in cities, and they are very comfortable with specific discriminations against rural people that have been institutionalized in China's employment and welfare systems since Mao's time. Some even look down on business people, especially the rural industrialists who have made China boom in recent decades. This ideology lasts mainly because it justifies the continuation in power of technocratic intellectuals who support each other. China's developmental changes will eventually make this political hauteur outdated. Unless China's elite is unlike any other that has been previously seen in history, some of its leading members will change their minds, become democrats, and thereby gain mandates from most of the population to govern in a more stable, less coercive, less punishment-oriented, more proveably representative fashion.

The SARS experience at least temporarily reduced the PRC elite's dislike of news transparency and distance from the "masses." Opining differently, however, Sunanda K. Datta-Ray of Nanyang Technological University speculates that SARS was a "setback for democracy."[52] He suggests, with some anti-Western venom but without benefit of evidence, that democratic

---

[51] On the comparative politics of this, see the classic analysis by Dankwart Rustow, "Transitions to Democracy: Toward a Dynamic Model," *Comparative Politics* 2: 3 (1970), pp. 337–363.
[52] Sunanda K. Datta-Ray, "A Setback for Democracy?" *International Herald Tribune*, June 2, 2003, p. 6. Datta-Ray, a distinguished former editor in India, is not Singaporean; but Singaporeans with Hindu surnames can be especially voluble elitists, perhaps because they are neither Chinese nor Muslim.

governments would have to oppose the quarantines that are necessary to maintain community health, and that incidents such as the riots at Tianjin clinics are excellent examples of democracy. They were actually examples of popular resentment against high-handed bureaucrats, who would be more efficient and politically stronger if they had clear mandates from a majority of the people. As for quarantines, governments with individualist and communitarian ideologies alike imposed or failed to impose them. Data from places as different as Toronto, Singapore, the Philippines, New York City, Vietnam, Taiwan, and Beijing clearly show that success against SARS depended on the timing of quarantines, not on the elites' preferred political philosophies. Singaporean illiberalism is easily justifiable, on a local basis, insofar as it prevents the political mobilization of Muslims against Chinese or vice-versa. "Racial" politics would pose a mortal threat to such a rich city-state of 4 m., so close to Indonesia that has a population fifty times as large, with a tiny Chinese minority owning most of the nonstate wealth. Unarticulated public apprehensions in Singapore's truly dangerous environment help legitimate an authoritarian regime, just as competitive elections would.[53] But these understandable reasons for illiberal hierarchy in Singapore's situation become ridiculous when applied to China, a country 300 times as populous in a context that is not ethnically challenged. Elites in the city-state strain their credibility, when they present policies that are sensible in their highly unusual context as if sensible everywhere.

Some Singapore spokespeople claim universal validity for hierarchal "Asian values," conflating Chinese with Muslim values as if everybody else were too stupid to notice the difference, and neglecting both populism in traditional Asia and elitism in the traditional West. The generalization (not the local policy against "racism") is another official fib. An unexplored problem for Singapore is that this discourse is warmly welcomed among Beijing elitists, who want to ignore the differences in national contexts and to suggest, against most of the evidence of their eyes, that anti-democracy is the key to prosperity everywhere. Singaporeans tend to underestimate the power of their own

---

[53] If the dangers nearby justify People's Action Party authoritarianism, so do habits such as the regime's great care in recruiting very smart technocrats. Periodic elections are held, albeit under rules that prevent unmediated popular power. At least the leaders rethink their policies, when oppositionists get as much as one-third of the general vote.

Not to put too fine a point on it, there are a lot of snobs in Beijing.

example among China's intellectuals. What's worse, they misjudge Singapore's own long-term interest, which is to encourage the rise of a PRC elite that condones less use of government violence. Acceptance of an elite's right to be brutal is dangerous for Singapore, above all in Indonesia, where state violence may later be turned against the rich Chinese minority.

Comparative evidence from most countries suggests that a democracy in China would soon or already be likely to survive very sturdily, *if* elites there brought themselves to channel their disputes through liberal mechanisms. The problem is that the PRC elite, for the most part, is still opposed to democracy. Not to put too fine a point on it, there are a lot of snobs in Beijing. Experiences like SARS are changing that, albeit very slowly. Political snobbery runs big costs, in an increasingly complex society and economy.

This problem is not restricted to mainland China. Taiwan's elite once had a similarly paternalistic attitude, at least under Chiang Kai-shek. As Arthur Lerman wrote, the history of that time shows "the elite's intention to control associations closely and to ensure their primary orientation toward approved goals." [54] Visiting Taiwan, Samuel Huntington once said that, "Reflecting, perhaps, traditional Confucian commitments to order, formality, and decorum, many people here expressed concern about...disturbing consequences of democratization. I would like to reassure these people. In general, democracies are often unruly, but they are rarely unstable. History shows that in complex and developed societies, democratic governments are very stable." [55]

Adam Przeworski and his colleagues in comparative political science have made a massive statistical study of *Democracy and Development* in all countries. Many of the facts they have unearthed disprove socio-political assumptions

---

[54] Arthur J. Lerman, *Taiwan's Politics: The Provincial Assemblyman's World* (Washington: University Press of America, 1979), p. 212, quoted in Shelley Rigger, "Mobilizational Authoritarianism and Political Opposition in Taiwan," *Political Oppositions in Industrializing Asia*, Garry Rodan, ed. (London: Routledge, 1996), p. 302.

[55] Samuel P. Huntington, "Foreword," in *Political Change in Taiwan*, Cheng Tun-jen and Stephan Haggard, eds. (Boulder: Lynne Rienner, 1992), p. xiii.

common among Beijing intellectuals. For example, comparative data show that "the durability of dictatorships [by this term, they mean any authoritarian regime, including China's] is unaffected by income distribution." [56] Elitists in China think, to the contrary, that their well-ordered regime is threatened by the gaping differences of income that have emerged during reforms. They are wrong, however, presuming that a comparative framework is the best way to make such a prediction. They bemoan the coast-inland wealth gap on grounds that go beyond humanitarianism; they think it threatens their own rule; but they should, on the basis of Przeworski's exhaustive study, rest easier. They can continue to rule a China that contains egregious income differentials, if they wish to do so.

Many Chinese intellectuals say that democracy would make their government weaker. They now know a good deal about the strengths (and defects) of liberal countries, but the community of educated people especially in Beijing discourages many compatriots from looking at the very notion of political development. Like Americans who can see no cogency in foreign resentments of the U.S. and who disregard some good reasons for those resentments, many Chinese intellectuals ignore the evidence of their eyes about the strengths of democracies. This myopia is most pronounced in Beijing.

They think that authoritarian regimes are always strong and democratic ones must be indecisive, even though they would agree with the present author about some of the disastrous strong decisions that democratically elected leaders have in fact taken. In parts of China far from the capital, the problems of this view become obvious especially in times of unexpected shocks. In Hong Kong, for example, the *Basic Law* makes the Chief Executive weaker — not stronger, despite legal appearances — because he cannot constitutionally seek a popular mandate to make decisions that would reallocate major resources. He cannot speak credibly for a majority of the people, because he lacks the normal modern means of showing that most people approve him as their representative. He would be hemmed in by the constitution that was written to petrify rule by tycoons, even if he wished to act as a broader representative. Land values have fallen by two-thirds, and SARS further raises Hong Kong's economic costs; so the Government is severely strapped for funds. It has proposed a risibly small 1% tax increase, but it cannot solve its main current problem by

---

[56] Adam Przeworski *et al.*, *Democracy and Development*, p. 120.

usual means, raising rates to levels that are normal in countries with Hong Kong's GDP per capita. The anti-populist constitution, which cannot in practice be amended, is exquisitely designed to preserve the authoritarian status quo, even though the context has changed sharply. It prevents strong rule, because the ruler cannot rely on a public mandate.

The PRC government could face parallel problems in coming years, if China's economy slows considerably. Random shocks, e.g. economic or medical, can affect politics. Such events could push China's elite toward either democracy or dictatorship. Current PRC technocrats are a bit more diverse than before the November 2002 Party Congress. They are smart engineers, but distant from most people. They are likely to discover, perhaps are already beginning to discover, that they need more than intelligence and engineering to solve China's problems. They need enthusiasm and support from people who have gained a sense of ownership in policies. This sense comes from having approved them, as against alternatives. It requires elite respect for all the varied truths.

Secret Lying versus Public Candor

Official lying is a habit that public intellectuals, at least since Machiavelli in the West and ancient Legalists in China, have rationalized by overstating the difficulty of creating communal order or of solving collective action problems. In the United States, former students of Leo Strauss, a deceased political philosopher at the University of Chicago, have used what they thought they learned from him about "noble lies." Radical neoconservatives under George W. Bush have been beguiled by the notion that ordinary people might be disturbed by the truth. They think that prevarication serves stability, or at least that any politician must conceal aims in order to remain in power.[57] Deputy Defense Secretary Paul Wolfowitz, as well as Abram Shulsky in the Pentagon's Office of Special Plans, took Ph.D. degrees under Professor Strauss.

---

[57] This view relates to Nietzsche's existentialism. It has a fascinating link to the difference between Weber and Selznick outlined in a China book: Franz Schurmann, *Ideology and Organization in Communist China* (Berkeley: University of California Press, 1966). This is not to say, however, that Max Weber, or perhaps Leo Strauss, would unreservedly approve the contemporary neoconservatives. Strauss disapproved much of Machiavelli.

They are reported to believe that "the essential truths about human society and history should be held by an elite, and withheld from others who lack the fortitude to deal with truth." [58] Since they distrust wholly public discourse, they prevent themselves from distinguishing the truth from their personal biases. In the formally democratic United States, no less than in authoritarian China, such leaders think they know the public interest better than the public does. [59] The quiet distrust they engender among many is a response to their own snobbery.

This tradition of esoteric elitism goes back to Plato and stresses the conscious unmasking of truths-for-the-few. More public versions of such ruses are ideologies, whose deceptions are not perceived as such because they are vaguely thought to have positive effects (and usually also the moot effect of keeping a current elite in power). Karl Mannheim, the classic sociologist of knowledge, wrote that, "We begin to treat our adversary's views as ideologies only when we no longer consider them as calculated lies and when we sense in his total behavior an unreliability which we regard as a function of the social situation in which he finds himself." [60] These ideological fibs are just half-consciously perceived as defective in truth because of the communal consequences of belief in them. They are not all conservative. A suicide bomber, half-sure of attaining heaven because of violence, has this kind of notion as surely as a rightist Myanmar general does. Ideological lying can, however, often be distinguished from conscious fibs.

Official lying in the SARS crisis has been extensive, and it has continued despite sporadic admonitions from top leaders to stop it. Historical hiding of public disasters in China has sometimes, however, been much worse. One example deserves special attention because of its egregiousness. An all-time

---

[58] William Pfaff, "The Long Reach of Leo Strauss," *International Herald Tribune*, May 15, 2003, p. 6.

[59] The cases of Wolfowitz and Shulsky, as of their associates Charles Feith and Richard Perle who apparently did not study with Strauss, are odd because their documentable past biases have favored Likud policies for "Greater Israel," a country different from America, whose security their main public posts suggest they should be serving. Facts about the links to Likud are at <http://www.antiwar.com/orig/lind1.html>. Likud policies (as distinct from policies of Israel's Labor Party or Peace Now groups, for example) together with U.S. aid and support for them are obvious among the factors that have clearly reduced the security of Americans, and could do so further in the future.

[60] Karl Mannheim, *Ideology and Utopia* (London: Routledge, 1936), p. 54.

world record for studious failure to publish news was set after the Tangshan earthquake of 1976, in which 250,000 people died. In terms of lives lost, this was the worst urban earthquake ever. It was not an easy time to gather information. Two Xinhua correspondents from Beijing, Zhang Guangyou and Luan Zhongxin, rushed to Tangshan in an overland jeep, saw people frantically trying to dig out roughly 70,000, who were still alive but trapped in building cave-ins, and interviewed cadres who reported that at least 10,000 coal miners must have been buried alive. Using a military wireless telephone (since the quake had cut all other forms of communication), these two reporters successfully filed their story, back to their editor in Beijing. It was never published. It might, after all, have distracted public attention from the officially vital news of mid-1976 (the grand successes of class struggle against Deng Xiaoping). It was not treated as proper news, since it might have diverted people's minds from ideas that the political elite of that time deemed more important.[61]

Popular disgust at officials, springing from a rich history of remembered lies and corruptions, has now been adapted to the current medical crisis. Reports have come of a popular joke: "The CCP can't stop wining and dining, yet SARS has done it; the CCP can't stop travel at official expense, yet SARS has done it; the CCP can't stop the mountains of documents and seas of meetings, yet SARS has done it; the CCP can't stop prostitution, yet SARS has done it...."[62] A Beijing taxi driver claimed, "The government's all just a bunch of gangsters."[63] That overstates the case, of course, but it may be as perceptive as most factional analysis because it takes into account an overall consonance of interest among elitists: the impulse to keep the vast majority of people out of political decisions.

In China, as in the West, some intellectuals are less disdainful. Zi Zhongyun, an eminent diplomatic historian and long-time Party member who is retired from the Chinese Academy of Social Sciences, remarked to a TV interviewer that, "The Chinese people can't be blamed for being in a panic about SARS,

---

[61] See Jing Jun, "The Working Press in China," unpublished paper sent to the author, 1985, p. 21.

[62] Personal communication from a Hong Kong reporter, whom this author thanks.

[63] Report from Rupert Wingfield-Hayes, BBC correspondent in Beijing, May 8, 2003, <http://news.bbc.co.uk/go/tr/fr/-/1/hi/world/asiapacific/3011739.stm>, May 20, 2003.

" They're lying. All the governments in Asia are lying. They're afraid of the money."

because they were lied to by Chinese officials."[64] Speaking on the anniversary of the May 4 Movement, she criticized Yan Fu (1854–1921), a famous early "modernizer" who nonetheless thought that the Chinese people should be denied democracy until they became better educated. Dr. Zi implied this is no political excuse for failing to educate them, by telling them the truth.

Another downside of official lying is that many people catch on to it very quickly. If elites alienate their potential support by being found telling conscious falsehoods, the reaction can be violently bitter. A Taichung, Taiwan, doctor commented on the official report that there was just a single confirmed SARS case in his city by saying that: "They're lying. All the governments in Asia are lying. They're afraid of the money."[65]

When local farmers realized that the government planned to use a school building as a quarantine quarters near the rural town of Chagugang, Tianjin, they wrecked the building. When a similar plan emerged in Tianjin's urban Hongqiao District during late April and early May, local riots and blockades stopped that arrangement. Similar reports came from Chongqing Municipality, Heping Hospital in Beijing, and Xiande in Zhejiang. An unelected government may have police, and it may have plans that actually serve the public interest, while nonetheless lacking a majority mandate to countervail local groups that can organize their own forces to insist that problems be fixed "not in my back yard."

Prevarication and political waffling has certainly not been a monopoly of Chinese in the SARS crisis. The World Health Organization, which must get along with governments, has also given the impression of having been influenced by political not just epidemiological considerations. The Mayor of Toronto implied this with great force on global television. WHO sent a small

---

[64] Interview on CCTV 9, May 4, 2003, 9:00 a.m. China time.
[65] When pressed with further questions, he agreed that Singapore "might not be lying very much" but believed that "for economic reasons, just about every other country in the region is lying through their teeth." April 13, 2003 posting by Tony Pace on the "Graphs and Models of the SARS Epidemic" website, at <http://www.sarswatch.org>, seen May 18, 1983.

delegation to investigate SARS in Taiwan, but these doctors saw no high officials because of PRC allergies to anything that resembles diplomacy on the island. Zhang Dejiang, the Guangdong party secretary, who repressed crucial early news about SARS but is reportedly Jiang Zemin's protégé, avoided dismissal in part because a WHO team visiting Guangdong gave an effusive report of cooperation by his network in its investigations of the province where the bug was born.

Fabrications have sometimes emerged from old bureaucratic habits and categories. If SARS patients in military hospitals of Beijing were soldiers, their household registrations (*hukou*) were in the army, not in any locality. So legally, they were not "in Beijing." Such an explanation for underreporting was publicly unpresentable, of course, but the inertia of bureaucratic and military habits clearly contributed to the SARS crisis.

At least through mid-May 2003, the reported data on SARS from Shanghai were lies (if those from elsewhere in China were true), because national standards for defining the disease were waived in that city. Shanghai is so important in terms of state revenues, it was allowed to avoid confirming a patient has having SARS until definite contact with a previously confirmed victim of the disease was established. A person on a death bed in Shanghai might clearly have atypical pneumonia, but would not be counted as having it until the place, time, and mode of transmission were recorded. Less restrictive criteria, approved by the WHO, applied in all other cities. This patent obfuscation "reduced" SARS in China's largest tax base. International officials protested, but by the time of this writing it was still not clear that the Shanghai medical authorities would have to conform to a standard definition of the disease, such as the epidemiologists surely needed.

Modern technology and international pressures deeply affected both the course of the epidemic and the politics surrounding it. Dr. Jiang Yanyong's e-mail abroad, discussed above, brought vital home truths back home to China. Hong Kong officials were not free to chastise the PRC government for its midwinter furtiveness that had let the epidemic get out of hand, but many other people in Hong Kong were not too shy to blame Communist secrecy. The Hong Kong Government Health Department was embarrassed by an independent webmaster (at www.sosick.org) into putting out its own daily information about the building locations of SARS cases (at www.info.gov.hk/dh/ap.htm). Apparently following this example, the PRC Health Ministry

Singapore Prime Minister Goh's cancellation of his trip to Beijing "on doctor's orders" was a sharp wake-up call for the new group of technocrats installed in the PRC.

then provided, on the internet each day, an updated map of the geographical distribution of reported SARS in China.[66]

International pressure to know the truth was crucial, from the very start of this epidemic to the time of its control, in the partial reduction of lying. Global impulses to transparency came from official sources, not just unofficial ones. Early in the epidemic, foreign leaders' criticisms of China, especially from Southeast Asia, made headlines. Singapore Prime Minister Goh's cancellation of his trip to Beijing "on doctor's orders" was a sharp wake-up call for the new group of technocrats installed in the PRC. This was quickly followed by Philippine President Arroyo's cancellation of a scheduled National People's Congress delegation, which was to have been headed by NPC head Wu Bangguo, to Manila; SARS dangers were explicit as the reason for the cancellation.[67] Statements from WHO and from ASEAN also soon criticized China for its mid-winter delay in reporting SARS, which was the most important human factor creating the epidemic. When problems become complex, as they do in modern times, it is helpful to have many monitors of them.

Conclusion: Serving the People versus Serving the Elite

Some Chinese intellectuals hoped that the epidemic might improve their country's governance. As Shanghai Normal University historian Xiao Gongqin

---

[66] See <http://www.supermap.com/sars>, May 19, 2003.

[67] Arroyo was also angry with the Hong Kong Government, which in its current budget crisis had announced a special new tax on Filipina amahs, the main English teachers of Hong Kong's middle-class children and the poorest large group in town. If philosopher John Rawls is right that the least advantaged people ought to be helped first, this Government was doing the diametric opposite of right.

said, "I think this disaster will make China's leaders more modest.... Everything seemed to be going so smoothly, and that allowed us to neglect our systemic shortcomings. This crisis is forcing everyone to reflect on those shortcomings. It will sharpen people's critical sense." The mishandling of the epidemic, according to a party official, was "a huge shock to the entire party. You can sense this at internal meetings, where the atmosphere has changed and people are expressing criticisms more freely. The SARS epidemic is forcing us to rethink the whole theoretical framework for our government that was developed under Jiang Zemin." [68] Whatever that framework might have been, among some intellectuals there is now perhaps a more specific interest in liberalizing it.

Party conservatives used this event for their purposes, too. Ignoring that the authoritarian tendency to ration truth had allowed the virus to get out of control originally, they suggested that quarantines would not have been possible under any other form of government. While media attention was focused on SARS, Chinese police clamped down on labor activists. Also, Huang Qi, webmaster of a site for information about missing persons (including dissidents whom the state may have caused to disappear), had been arrested in June 2000 and in August 2001 secretly convicted of "subverting state sovereignty"; he was sentenced to prison in May 2003.[69] The SARS scare was a time when the authorities arrested oppositionists, apparently thinking nobody would notice.

Change is difficult for reformers because of inertia in any large Leninist (or other) system. Soviet leaders who wanted to save their state by modernizing it were constrained by the institutions and habits that preceded them.[70] To some extent this was an old problem. Lenin himself understood, only at the very end of his life in his last letters, that Russian traditions (embodied in Stalin's style of rule) would negate the revolution for which Lenin knew he had sacrificed many others' lives.[71] Half a century later, Gorbachev faced the

---

[68] "A New Era in China as SARS Takes Dazzle out of the Future," p. 1.

[69] Verna Yu, "China Webmaster Gets Five Years," *South China Morning Post*, May 19, 2003, p. 4.

[70] See Philip G. Roeder, *Red Sunset: The Failure of Soviet Politics* (Princeton: Princeton University Press, 1993).

[71] See V.I. Lenin, "On Bureaucracy," "Letter to the Congress," "Better Fewer, But Better," and "Last Letters," in Robert C. Tucker, ed., *The Lenin Anthology* (New York: Norton, 1975), pp. 714–718, 725–728.

China will continue to be mismanaged until the government comes closer to the people, that is, until Chinese intellectuals realize they live in a large country that requires many kinds of leaders.

less severe late-Communist form of this problem: "We are now, as it were, going through the school of democracy afresh. We are learning. Our political culture is still inadequate. Our standard of debate is inadequate; our ability to respect the point of view of even our friends and comrades — even that is inadequate." [72]

"Democratic centralism" can become at least as arthritic as other forms of democracy, although many quasi-Leninists remaining in the world deny this. Gorbachev as head of the USSR did not hear about the Chernobyl disaster until more than 24 hours later, and that was a far more sudden and incontrovertible crisis than the quiet emergence of a hard-to-diagnose fever in a distant province. Many intellectuals' overestimation of the efficiency of Leninist bureaucracies is a phenomenon that deserves more study.[73]

Chinese politics are now somewhat fluid. The CCP "ceases to be a party of devoted cadres [and] is evolving into an aggregation of heterogeneous interests, a catch-all party managed by professional party workers." [74] (These words were actually used to describe the KMT of the 1980s, but they apply just as well across the Strait at present.) The SARS crisis and other socioeconomic problems of the future might prove to be a partial "opening" for the Chinese political system. Many western journalists and scholars implicitly understate the complexity of China's structure. The barriers to good communication between localities and the central government remain formidable. SARS spread partly because of organizational failure in a huge polity run by an anti-populist

---

[72] Gorbachev is quoted in Ronald Inglehart, *Modernizations and Post-Modernizations*, p. 162.

[73] An example may be recent revision of the main ideas in Andrew Walder, *Communist Neo-Traditionalism: Work and Authority in Chinese Industry* (Berkeley: University of California Press, 1986).

[74] Cheng Tun-jen, "Taiwan in Democratic Transition," in J. Morley, ed., *Driven by Growth: Political Change in the Asia-Pacific Region* (Armonk: Sharpe, 1993), p. 215.

elite. China will continue to be mismanaged until the government comes closer to the people, that is, until Chinese intellectuals realize they live in a large country that requires many kinds of leaders.

There will surely be future epidemics out of China *and* other countries, although it is impossible to predict the exact traits of any upcoming pathogens. The Pearl River Delta has long been famous for producing "Hong Kong" or "Asian" flus.[75] In fact, however, any part of the planet that has people in close proximity to other mammals and birds can provide a site for germs to jump from those species to *Homo sapiens*. Despite his name, *homo* is often not as bright as he thinks he is. Would humans, for example, be able to contain the pandemic of a germ that might have many of these traits: as easily caught as most coronaviruses (such as cause colds), as genetically stable as SARS (so that it would not mutate into less virulent forms), as deadly as Ebola (which had a nine-tenths mortality rate), but with slow incubation (even a fraction of the period HIV takes, during which time it can spread widely)? No such bug has appeared, fortunately. But it could. *Homo* might get his act together and become more *sapiens* quickly, because a future germ with some of these characteristics would, in the current age, take global airplane trips as easily as SARS did — and could be far more dangerous.

If atypical pneumonia helps the human community develop an iron-clad norm that new diseases absolutely must be reported in public just as soon as they are suspected, it may prove to be a blessing in much disguise. If elites continue to distrust ordinary citizens so deeply that they continue to suppress free flows of information about public problems, however, such problems can become worse. Honesty really is the best policy, even though an old motto says so.

---

[75] Because of SARS, Guangdong markets were reorganized; so outbreaks of new germs there are less likely. Beijing bans on pets and Singapore executions of stray cats were rituals that showed ferocious wills to majesty in those states, but no evidence suggests these actions affected SARS. Socio-political purification rites, notably against cats, have also appeared in the West; see Robert Darnton, *The Great Cat Massacre and Other Episodes in French Cultural History* (New York: Basic Books, 1984).

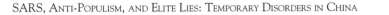

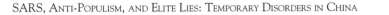

Lynn T. White III

Prof. Lynn T. White III teaches about China and comparative development at Princeton University in the Woodrow Wilson School, Politics Department, and East Asian Studies Program. He has written four books on political history since 1949 in Shanghai and the Yangzi Delta, two edited tomes on comparative politics and social policy, and articles for *China Quarterly*, *Journal of Asian Studies*, *American Political Science Review*, *Asian Survey*, and other journals. His interest in SARS arose because he was on research leave in Hong Kong when the bug struck that city, working at Hong Kong University's Centre of Asian Studies with support from the Chiang Ching-kuo Foundation. Lynn is solely to blame for all his views.

Correspondence to: Prof. Lynn T. White, E-mail: lynn@Princeton.EDU.

4

Baptism by Storm: The SARS Crisis' Imprint on China's New Leadership

by *Christopher A. McNally*

1. Introduction

The Chinese leadership transition that was completed in early March represented the most orderly, peaceful, and rule-bound political succession in the history of the People's Republic of China. It consisted of the transfer of power from third generation leaders with Jiang Zemin at their helm to fourth generation leaders headed by Hu Jintao. The smooth succession symbolized to the world that China was coming of age, adding to past successes such as winning the right to host the 2008 Olympics and fostering blooming relations with the United States and other great powers.

However, as the leadership transition was unfolding in the cavernous Hall of the People in early March 2003, a new mysterious and sneaky danger lurked

Miscalculation and a long held penchant to bury unfavorable information and statistics in China led to a news blackout about the nature and extent of the SARS epidemic.

under the veneer of China's recent successes. Severe Acute Respiratory Syndrome (SARS) had already infected hundreds of people in Guangdong province and was starting to spread rapidly to other Chinese provinces and abroad. Miscalculation and a long held penchant to bury unfavorable information and statistics in China led to a news blackout about the nature and extent of the SARS epidemic. The viral disease was therefore able to penetrate deep into Beijing, China's cultural and political center. Its rapid spread throughout the spring of 2003 forced China's new fourth generation leaders to face their first major test within only a few weeks of taking power. Indeed, the epidemic jolted China's polity and society in ways not seen since the 1989 Tiananmen incident.

In this essay I will draw two related though distinct inferences from China's handling of the SARS crisis. First, analyzing the new leadership's reaction to the SARS epidemic opens an ideal window into examining the present nature and logic of China's party-state. This analysis, which will be presented in the first part of the essay, shows that China's political system constitutes an amalgam of old and new.[1] Maoist mass mobilization coexists with modern management techniques and public relations exercises. This relationship, however, is an uneasy one. It must be gradually resolved by the Chinese party-state's continuous adaptation to new social and economic circumstances.

Second, the SARS crisis holds the potential to shape the political orientation and policies of the fourth generation leadership in the near future. The shock to China's political and social system created by SARS is further liable to cause a reorientation of the country's political economy. This

---

[1] See David Shambaugh, "Introduction: The Evolving and Eclectic Modern Chinese State," in David Shambaugh, ed. *The Modern Chinese State* (Cambridge: Cambridge University Press, 2000), p. 1.

70

reorientation, though, will be evolutionary rather than revolutionary. The second part of this essay will elucidate three areas in which change is most likely: transparency, accountability, and social justice.

Furthermore, the SARS epidemic, if it does not persist for much beyond the second quarter of 2003, is likely to strengthen the hand of the two core leaders among the fourth generation — Hu Jintao and Wen Jiabao. It is also likely to prod these leaders to make incremental changes to the country's political economy. The shift in public sentiment following the SARS crisis, especially widespread disillusionment with the present political system among Chinese intellectuals and party insiders, might act to imbue momentum to the pace of change.

2. China's Handling of SARS: The Anatomy of a Party-State

As the first cases of SARS appeared in Guangdong in late fall 2002, medical practitioners and local officials knew little about what kind of disease had struck.[2] However, as the disease spread, many local doctors became alarmed and reported in early January 2003 strange clusters of pneumonia to Guangdong provincial authorities. Experts sent out concluded that they faced a type of pneumonia of previously unknown cause. Although some effective health measures were taken at the local level, the virus spread and moved on to the provincial capital of Guangzhou. Provincial officials notified central disease control and health authorities in early February, but what the content of this information was and how central officials reacted is still unknown.[3] What is known is that panic spread more rapidly than SARS via text messaging, Internet chat rooms and word of mouth in the Pearl River Delta. On February 10, provincial authorities made a public announcement. However, subsequently authorities instituted a far-reaching news blackout.

The motivation for this news blackout originated from a variety of sources, all of which are tied to the culture and structure of China's political system.

---

[2] For an excellent initial recount of the spreading of SARS see Elisabeth Rosenthal, "From China's Provinces, A Crafty Germ Spreads," *New York Times Internet Edition*, April 27, 2003.
[3] Josephine Ma, "Guangdong Reported on the Outbreak in February," *South China Morning Post Internet Edition*, May 21, 2003.

Throughout the history of the People's Republic many sensitive public health matters have been treated as state secrets.

The initial outbreak of panic in the Pearl River Delta around February 12 is likely to have persuaded Guangdong officials that to come clean on the new epidemic would create more panic and the potential for social chaos. The reaction of officials was also driven by an embedded culture of secrecy and elitism in China's party-state. Throughout the history of the People's Republic many sensitive public health matters have been treated as state secrets for fear of causing social instability and shedding a bad light on government health policies.

In addition, officials are likely to have opted for secrecy due to a concern for their own political wellbeing. Local and provincial officials in China are evaluated on a variety of standards pertaining to the conditions in their localities, most of which emphasize economic development and social stability. Reporting openly on the outbreak of SARS in Guangdong would have affected foreign investment and international economic transactions, a scenario the leaders of China's export powerhouse wanted to avoid. The outbreak of SARS in Guangzhou also occurred just around the Lunar New Year. Any large-scale panic or fear would have directly influenced consumption during this most important Chinese holiday.

Finally, once figures for Guangdong were released in late March, these suggested that cases diminished throughout March. Perhaps officials in Guangdong thought that they could bring the disease under control during February, thus presenting a bright and stable picture of their province to the outside world.

The cover-up of SARS backfired massively. After February 21, SARS spread to Hong Kong and then internationally. It also gained a foothold in China's capital and several northern provinces, most notably Shanxi and Inner Mongolia. Despite the rapid spread of SARS, China's government kept the news blackout intact and actively tried to conceal the extent of the outbreak. In April, international pressure grew, a World Health Organization (WHO) team announced that they doubted the reported figures for Beijing's sick, and Jiang Yanyong, a retired People's Liberation Army doctor, exposed government efforts to cover up the SARS crisis in Beijing's military hospitals. As in Guangdong, mouth-to-mouth word and information transmitted via text messaging and the Internet started to create popular pressure and panic. Reports have also noted that SARS started to directly affect the Communist Party elite in Beijing, even infecting employees in the Zhongnanhai leadership compound.[4]

By April 20, the government made the decision that to continue the cover up would create more damage than to come clean. The U-turn in government policy was stunning. The health minister and the mayor of Beijing were fired, ostensibly for policy failures, and the media and party were ordered to be absolutely transparent what concerned the extent and nature of the epidemic. The government further pledged to actively cooperate with the WHO and put Vice-premier Wu Yi, a technocratic troubleshooter in the style of Zhu Rongji, in charge of the health system.

In essence, the country was put on a war footing. In a manner harking back to Maoist times, the party and media mass mobilized society into confronting the SARS crisis. Airwaves were rapidly filled with advice about hygiene and pleas to remain calm. Media outlets also portrayed the battle against SARS as a test of the whole nation, exhorting people to rally around the communist leadership to overcome the country's hardship. In another instance of Maoist mobilization, Beijing authorities flattened an old Communist Party resort to build a thousand-bed hospital to house SARS patients. In just over a week, a crew of 4000 construction workers laboring around the clock realized what is probably the world's fastest construction of a major health facility. Perhaps most telling was the mobilization of the traditional neighborhood committees — the Communist states tentacles into urban society — to fight SARS. Mainly elderly residents investigated individual households in their neighborhood to ascertain that there are no SARS cases and barred outsiders from entering compounds to forestall the spreading of the disease.[5]

Both the initial cover up and the subsequent mass mobilization of society to fight SARS tell us much about the nature and logic of China's contemporary

---

[4] Joseph Kahn, "SARS Reaches Near Top of Chinese Communist Hierarchy," *New York Times Internet Edition*, April 30, 2003.
[5] "Neighborhood Watches Join SARS Battle," *South China Morning Post Internet Edition*, May 16, 2003.

| Both the initial cover up and the subsequent mass mobilization of society to fight SARS tell us much about the nature and logic of China's contemporary party-state.

party-state. The features that emanate present an amalgam of old and new, imported and indigenous. Five features are particularly noteworthy:

Fragmented and Decentralized Governance

The Chinese state has moved from being a highly centralized, coercive and authoritarian state in the Mao era to a more diffuse entity. Specifically, the reform period has unleashed several waves of decentralization, further fragmenting structures of authority.[6] These trends are especially pronounced in the nation's healthcare system, a perfect arena for analyzing the effects of China's reforms. Before the reform period hospitals were administered by a variety of institutions, including local governments, state enterprises, schools and the military. Although standards varied and were often minimal in the countryside, the provision of free healthcare was quite universal in the pre-reform era.

As decentralization and commercialization increased in the 1980s and 1990s, the different administrative jurisdictions in hospital management were left mainly to their own devices. This created a fragmented hospital system with little provincial-level or central coordination. Unequal access to healthcare also became a defining feature, since in richer jurisdictions local administrative units were able to invest in healthcare, while in poorer areas the healthcare system either became privatized or disintegrated. Overall, government investment in healthcare has been minimal.

The mainland's recent establishment of new disease-control institutions at the central and provincial levels has not been able to overcome the

---

[6] See on this point Kenneth Lieberthal and Michel Oksenberg, eds., *Policy Making in China — Leaders, Structures and Processes* (Princeton: Princeton University Press, 1988).

Unequal access to healthcare also became a defining feature.

fragmentation in medical care management. Especially timely information provision on new diseases is hampered because local doctors first report to local disease control centers. The provincial officials who appoint the top staff of these centers can interfere in their work and forestall information flows to central authorities. Ultimately, this is an effect of the *tiaotiao* / *kuaikuai* organization of China's administrative system, whereby officials are appointed by local governments but functionally responsible to their superior organization at a higher level of government. Conflicts of interest are unavoidable under this system, undermining transparent and effective reporting mechanisms in many areas of governance.

The fragmentation of governance also became apparent in the aftermath of the government's U-turn in dealing with the SARS crisis. Although the government made it clear that it wanted commerce and trade flows to continue freely, many local governments started to stop buses, trucks and trains from infected areas such as Guangdong and Beijing. Villages around Beijing erected makeshift barricades and posted sentinels to keep strangers out, while many localities imposed excessively restrictive quarantine rules, effectively barring any visitors from affected areas.[7] Perhaps most tellingly, the central government's exhortations that migrant laborers should stay put fell on deaf ears. After the April 20 announcements a flood of rural migrants fled the capital, raising the specter of spreading SARS into the countryside.

Insufficient Checks and Balances

The paucity of effective and open reporting concerning social and economic problems is aggravated by the lack of external and internal checks. In some areas the Chinese government has sought to strengthen central information collecting institutions, such as the State Statistical Bureau. However, China's

---

[7] Christopher Bodeen, "Chinese Villagers Barricade Against SARS — Many Stay Home for May Day Holiday," *Washington Post Internet Edition*, May 1, 2003, 1:10 PM.

political system is still highly stratified and top-down. Local officials can easily divert bottom-up information flows and within the political system there is limited room for dissent. The culture of secrecy in China, whereby even mundane information is categorized as a state secret, aggravates this situation.

Perhaps the most severe shortcoming lies in the overall management of public information. On all sensitive issues, especially matters pertaining to national security and social stability, China's media outlets receive instructions from propaganda departments. Sometimes media restrictions amount merely to a light touch, providing some room for independent reporting. In other cases, central and local propaganda departments can gag the media. As the initial handling of SARS in Guangdong shows, once leaders decide an issue is too sensitive, they can order a virtual media blackout.

In recent years, the role of the media as an independent channel for information has increased. Because local government leaders regularly cheat the central government in forestalling or falsifying information flows, the central government has begun to encourage a degree of media openness, one of the only means for central policy makers to obtain reliable information. Yet, the problem of local government leaders and propaganda officials being able to interfere in what is reported remains. Both the problems of fragmented governance and insufficient checks and balances on government behavior thus converge. Crisis situations are covered up and allowed to develop to hardly manageable proportions.

Mass Campaigns and Leninist Organization

The above two features of the Chinese political system have pointed to its drawbacks. However, the centralized top-down nature of the party-state and its control over information are also potent weapons, weapons that have been

The paucity of effective and open reporting concerning social and economic problems is aggravated by the lack of external and internal check.

Not only did the media report candidly on the extent of SARS and give health and epidemiological advice, it also exhorted the Chinese to rally around the leadership and overcome the national hardship.

put to their ultimate use in dealing with the SARS crisis. As soon as the government decided to come clean, the nation's propaganda apparatus and media organizations sprung into full action. Not only did the media report candidly on the extent of SARS and give health and epidemiological advice, it also exhorted the Chinese to rally around the leadership and overcome the national hardship. The government's massive failure to deal initially with the SARS crisis was turned into a national cry for unity. As a People's Daily headline, taking an obvious cue from the reaction to the events of September 11 in the United States, put it: "In crisis, we stand together." [8]

The government's reaction was not confined to the media. The party apparatus as a whole sprung into action, mobilizing various parts of society to face the crisis. As noted above, neighborhood committees were revitalized, new hospitals constructed and the military brought into action. One report even stated that the government deployed 5 million reservists and militia to 50,000 villages in Hebei to educate rural Chinese on SARS.[9] In a similar fashion, military medical personnel were mobilized to join the anti-SARS fight in Beijing and other cities. For anybody following the events in China, the mobilization of people and resources unfolding after April 20 was nothing less than astounding.

To back up this mass mobilization, the government also resorted to some draconian measures. Over 10,000 people were put in quarantine in Beijing, new regulations with stiff penalties drawn up, and the threat of the death penalty invoked for anybody who knowingly spread SARS. The top-down

---

[8] Josephine Ma, "Mainland Media Faces Major Test of its Credibility," *South China Morning Post Internet Edition*, April 25, 2003.

[9] "Alternative SARS Remedies Cause for Government Concern," *Stratfor.com (Strategic Forecasting LLC)*, May 19, 2003, p. 2.

Leninist system was also put to effective use to create better information flows. Party edicts made clear that no secrecy concerning local SARS outbreaks would be tolerated. As a result, cadre incentives were shifted overnight to invoke high degrees of transparency and timely reporting what concerned the disease. As one Beijing resident put it: "The government can really get things done when it wants to."[10]

New Society

The above feature demonstrates that the Chinese party-state is still effective in dealing with emergencies and crises. It continues to possess the political and social tools to mobilize society, change cadre incentives and put an immense amount of resources to rapid use. Other recent examples of this effective handling of socioeconomic threats includes the crackdown on smuggling led by Zhu Rongji in the late 1990s and the suppression of the Falun Gong movement. Where the party-state fares worse is in effective day-to-day governance. Indeed, the rapid changes in socioeconomic conditions unfolding in China over the past 25 years have created a disjuncture between the day-to-day governance capabilities of the party-state and social conditions.

Economic reforms have made society much more mobile. An estimated 150 to 200 million rural residents are considered surplus labor, unable to find employment in the fields. Many of these therefore travel throughout the country in search of work, most of which is located in the big cities. In addition, many urban residents have become highly mobile, flying between provinces for business or pleasure. This higher mobility has allowed SARS to spread rapidly within China and also made the task of containing the disease more difficult. Most importantly, social and political governance in China has not caught up with this reality.

Due to the residency (*hukou*) system, rural laborers in big cities are unable to take advantage of the social infrastructure available to urban residents. As the government came clean on SARS in late April, the knee-jerk reaction of

---

[10] Erick Eckholm, "As Toll Mounts, Chinese Officials Try to Calm Panicky Public," *New York Times Internet Edition*, May 1, 2003.

Rural migrants feared that if they fell sick they would be unable to obtain medical care and other support in the cities. The system of governance therefore amplified the risks of spreading SARS into the countryside.

rural residents fearing contamination was to immediately head back to the villages. Ultimately, this was a natural reaction, since rural migrants feared that if they fell sick they would be unable to obtain medical care and other support in the cities. The system of governance therefore amplified the risks of spreading SARS into the countryside.

The old style of governance has also become less effective due to new modes of telecommunication and the internationalization of China's economy. After the Guangdong authorities made their announcement about SARS on February 10, news spread rapidly via text messaging. The news blackout and the arrest of five people for using text messaging to spread rumors contained this initial burst of information sharing.[11] In view of the government's cover up of the SARS outbreak, it is highly likely that text messaging will become an even more important means of sharing information in the future. Text messaging is particularly fit for this, since unlike the Internet, it remains unregulated by government authorities.

The internationalization of China is having similar effects. The increasing integration of China into the global economy can now more easily translate China's problems into global problems. Although the government initially resisted international pressure concerning SARS, the point at which the costs of a continued cover up exceeded the costs of coming clean arrived much earlier due to the immense shortfall China would have faced if international investors and traders left the country. Heeding international opinion has thus become a much more important feature of China's politics.

---

[11] Michael Jen-Siu, "Text Messaging Worries Authorities," *South China Morning Post Internet Edition*, February 19, 2003.

Finally, China's economic reforms have produced a burgeoning middle class in the major cities and coastal areas. The aspirations of this middle class have been partially hurt by the handling of the SARS crisis. At a minimum, disillusionment with the present political system is set to rise and move to the forefront of many urban residents' concerns. As one master's degree student at Beijing's Renmin University put it: "This is a problem of the system. Although China hasn't developed to the level of a democracy, the government ought to take responsibility for the livelihoods and health of its people." [12]

Partial Adaptation

Many western commentaries tend to point out that China's political system is anachronistic and unable to deal with new socioeconomic developments. As a *New York Times* commentary put it: "China's ossified political system is out of sync with China's globalized, market-driven economy." [13] This statement is only partially true. The Chinese party-state has started to adapt in quite significant ways to new social and economic realities. [14] The U-turn on SARS presents a variety of indicators on how the Chinese party-state is adjusting.

Although several commentators note that the firing of Zhang Wenkang, the health minister, and Meng Xuenong, the mayor of Beijing, might be tied to factional struggles, it is much more likely that the firing was a symbolic admission of the government's (though not the party's) failure to deal effectively with SARS. This has established a certain standard of accountability. In the place of these two officials, Premier Wen Jiabao anointed Vice-Premier Wu Yi to be in charge of the health system and Wang Qishan to become mayor of Beijing. Both of these officials have excelled at crisis management. Their appointment also signifies that the technocratic legacy

---

[12] Charles Hutzler and Peter Wonacott, "SARS Threatens to Impact Chinese Politics, Economy — Foreign Investors Step Back As Crisis Hampers Growth; Outrage Focuses on Beijing," *Asian Wall Street Journal*, April 30, 2003, p. A1.

[13] "Diagnosing SARS in China," *New York Times Internet Edition*, May 19, 2003.

[14] One recent academic argument along these lines is Andrew Nathan, "China's Changing of the Guard — Authoritarian Resilience," *Journal of Democracy*, Vol. 14, No. 1, January 2003, pp. 6–17. Several other contributors in this issue take a view contrary to Nathan's.

During Wen Jiabao's first visit abroad to a special summit called by the Association of Southeast Asian Nations and China to address the SARS crisis, he did an excellent job at bridging China's credibility gap.

of Zhu Rongji, which puts more emphasis on the ability of officials than on their factional associations, is likely to continue.

The government's public relations management capabilities have also improved considerably. During Wen Jiabao's first visit abroad to a special summit called by the Association of Southeast Asian Nations and China to address the SARS crisis, he did an excellent job at bridging China's credibility gap.[15] Within China the appointment of Wu Yi, one of the country's most popular politicians with men and women, has also had the effect to assure China's populace as well as foreign investors. Subsequent statements and actions by her have further assuaged concerns. For example, when she arrived in the city of Tianjin to examine SARS prevention measures, she immediately dialed the 120 SARS reporting hotlines to see whether it worked. After she received no answer, she barked at the local party secretary demanding he fix the situation immediately.[16]

China's party-state's gradual adaptation is also evident in the issuing of new Emergency Regulations on Sudden Outbreaks of Public Health Incidents.[17] Although stern in nature, the new regulations clearly spell out the responsibilities of local officials in disease prevention. Increasingly, therefore, the government is resorting to openly published and codified legal and administrative regulations to deal with social issues, a substantial improvement over internal party edicts.

---

[15] Nailene Chou Wiest, "Sound Start as Premier Presses the Right Buttons," *South China Morning Post Internet Edition*, May 1, 2003.

[16] John Pomfret, "In Crisis, China Turns to a Familiar Face," *Washington Post*, May 6, 2003, p. A17.

[17] BBC Worldwide Monitoring, "China's People's Daily Views 'Major Disaster' of SARS Epidemic," *BBC Monitoring Asia Pacific — Political*, May 12, 2003.

3. The SARS Crisis' Imprint on Fourth Generation Leadership

I examined in the above what the handling of the SARS crisis tells us about the nature of China's contemporary political system — the anatomy of the party-state. What emerged was a picture of a highly powerful party-state that nonetheless has increasing difficulties in dealing with the day-to-day management of new social and political phenomena. While the party-state still retains considerable capabilities to mobilize people and resources on a massive scale, it also is moving towards more open and regularized modes of governance. In short, the Chinese party-state is an amalgam of old and new, a hybrid that is transitioning from a Maoist mode of rule to a more modern, albeit still authoritarian style of governing society.

However, the perhaps most interesting aspect of how China handled the SARS crisis is not what it tells us about the present. More fascinating is whether the new leadership's reaction to the SARS outbreak allows us to discern new trends in China's polity. These trends are likely to be evolutionary in nature, unfolding slowly over the next five years. Isolating these new trends is also by necessity a speculative exercise. Nonetheless, I will venture to propose that there are three distinct areas in which we should expect change: transparency, accountability, and social justice.

Transparency

The government's U-turn and subsequent openness about SARS is in and of itself remarkable. After April 20 the party machinery immediately encouraged more open reporting and ordered officials at all levels to be honest and forthright with the conditions in their localities. The openness, though, was not complete. In Guangdong, officials are still only providing minimal information on how the initial outbreak unfolded. As a senior reporter with a party newspaper put it: "It doesn't matter if [President] Hu Jintao has ordered more transparency. As long as your immediate boss does not tell you to speak to the press, you don't do it." [18]

---

[18] Leu Siew Ying, "Media Being Kept in the Dark in Guangdong," *South China Morning Post Internet Edition*, May 12, 2003.

The degree of new media openness will thus be constrained. Highly sensitive political issues will continue to be out-of-bounds, while local officials will still repress media reporting on matters that might reflect badly on local conditions. In other words, the fragmented governance of China and the long-held penchant for secrecy in the Communist party-state will hardly vanish over night. Despite this, a new trend is clearly emerging.

Besides bold reporting on the SARS crisis, as for example by the *Caijing* magazine, other sociopolitical issues have been much more closely scrutinized since mid-April 2003. Most telling is the amount of information provided on an accident involving a People's Liberation Navy submarine in the Yellow Sea that killed 70 sailors. China's military has never before acknowledged such accidents. In this case, though, state-run television showed China's two senior leaders, President Hu Jintao and Jiang Zemin, meeting family members of those killed in the accident. Hu was quoted as saying that the accident should be seen as a way to prompt greater efforts at military modernization in China. As an expert on Chinese security at Fudan University, Shen Dingli, put it: "This whole affair is a breakthrough for openness."[19]

In a similar vein, a whole range of other issues has been put to greater scrutiny. In early May, China's Ministry of Labor and Social Security announced that it will soon broaden the definition of "unemployed" to include the underemployed, a long overdue move to increase the transparency of China's urban labor markets. And on May 16, Professor Wu Zhongmin from the Central Party School wrote in the *China Economic Times* that the government should adjust its poverty line and revise its poverty figures.[20] Overall, much more open calls for reforming the country's healthcare system and other social welfare functions have emerged in newspaper editorials. Although this could not be independently confirmed, one report even noted that the Chinese State Council was considering new regulations that will enshrine the people's "right to know" and impose disclosure obligations on officials.[21]

---

[19] John Pomfret, "Reports Show China Openness — Range of Detail in Sub Accident is Called 'Very Postitive Thing'," *Asian Wall Street Journal*, May 7, 2003, p. A4.

[20] Josephine Ma, "Scholar Scorns Mainland's Poverty Figures," *South China Morning Post Internet Edition*, May 17, 2003.

[21] Edith Terry, "Evolution, Not Revolution," *South China Morning Post Internet Edition*, April 26, 2003.

In sum, the government's failure to effectively contain SARS in the first few months of 2003 and the subsequent top-down imposition of open reporting unleashed a wave of greater transparency in China. It is likely that the government, once conditions return to normal, will attempt to reign in the forces it set free. However, Hu Jintao's and Wen Jiabao's legitimacy hinges to a considerable degree on continuing the trend towards greater government transparency. In essence, China's new fourth generation leaders will be walking a tightrope. Too much openness could stir social unrest and delegitimize the party-state. Too little openness could lead to widespread cynicism which could come back to haunt the leadership during the next crisis.

Accountability

With the firing of China's health minister and mayor of Beijing, Premier Wen Jiabao and President Hu Jintao took responsibility for handling the SARS crisis and installed two technocratic troubleshooters to directly deal with the epidemic. The actions of top government leaders constituted an implicit admission of fault. In fact, humbleness and forthrightness became the characteristics emanating from the leadership, both in national and international forums.

The promulgation of new regulations on the handling of disease incidents also constitutes an important step towards assigning clearer accountability. For instance, these regulations reinforce the responsibilities of provincial-level governments, stipulating that these must report to the State Council's administrative department for public health within one hour of receiving reports of epidemics and other sudden incidents. The regulations also lay down strict legal responsibilities for governments and government departments that conceal, put off reporting or lie about sudden outbreaks of diseases. Accountability is thus more clearly pinpointed.

Ultimately, pressures for enforcing greater accountability are likely to emanate via changes to the cadre management system. Recent studies have shown that this system has been quite adaptable throughout the reform period, increasing in some arenas the capacity of the central state to monitor and control lower level officials.[22] It is quite likely that over the coming few years the incentive systems for cadres will once again be adjusted, enforcing stricter standards of accountability that will be backed up by greater government transparency and media openness. The new incentive systems are also likely to move away from focusing on the single minded pursuit of economic development to emphasize more prominently issues of social justice.

Social Justice

Even before the SARS crisis erupted, China's two new top leaders, Hu Jintao and Wen Jiabao, started to focus on issues of social justice. Highly publicized trips to the herders of Inner Mongolia and the coal miners of Shanxi portrayed the two leaders as being concerned with the plight of China's poor and disadvantaged. Indeed, studies by the Central Party School and other think-tanks have shown an alarming increase of social inequalities in China, conditions that could easily lead to severe incidents of unrest and political opposition to Communist Party rule.

The SARS crisis has served to further highlight the conditions of social inequality in China. At a minimum, the crisis will accelerate plans to establish a bare-bones public healthcare system for rural residents. It will also lead to reforms of the country's disease reporting and response mechanisms. A much more consolidated and better-coordinated public health surveillance system is a necessity, since at present the regulatory functions of China's health system are in shambles. Vice-premier Wu Yi already announced in late April 2003 that the government plans to spend 3.5 billion Yuan to set up a nationwide health network to fight SARS and other medical emergencies.[23]

Overall, the minds of many Chinese will be more focused on issues of healthcare, cleanliness, and clean governance. Calls for nationwide healthcare reforms will certainly become stronger. However, healthcare reform will necessitate the provision of widely available health insurance, the

---

[22] Maria Edin, "State Capacity and Local Agent Control in China: CCP Cadre Management from a Township Perspective," *China Quarterly*, No. 173, March 2003.

[23] "Anti-SARS Health Network Established," *South China Morning Post Internet Edition*, April 26, 2003.

establishment of sustainable financing mechanisms for this insurance, and the construction of safety nets for the poor. All of these items require far reaching institutional reforms and large financial contributions by all levels of government. To what extent governments can marshal such funds is questionable. Fiscal decentralization has created severe budgetary constraints for local governments. Moreover, the Communist Party's commitment to use taxation as a tool for social redistribution is unlikely to be strong, since this will require much higher taxes for China's rich. The dilemma is that most of China's rich are private entrepreneurs, a segment of the population on which the party is relying more and more for economic growth and political support.

Despite these inherent political and institutional obstacles, the SARS crisis might serve as an impetus for gradual change in China. The crisis is already costing China dearly in economic and diplomatic terms. The internal legitimacy of the regime is also under greater pressure than at any time since the 1989 Tiananmen Square incident. As a response to these pressures, China's new leaders have undergone an image makeover. Hu Jintao and Wen Jiabao in particular are presenting a humane and kind face. At the end of the day, China's new leaders must follow through on their words. More resources for healthcare, substantial efforts at narrowing the gap between rich and poor, and a general movement away from the single-minded pursuit of economic growth to focus more on issues of social welfare and justice is thus likely.

IV. Conclusion

The SARS crisis has highlighted how the Chinese party-state combines in often uneasy fashion Maoist mass mobilization with modern methods of crisis management. From the vantage point of late May 2003, the measures taken by the Chinese government seem to have produced considerable success in

A general movement away from the single-minded pursuit of economic growth to focus more on issues of social welfare and justice is thus likely.

It is likely that once the SARS crisis passes, China will return to politics as usual. Nonetheless, the shock to China's political and social system created by SARS is liable to cause a reorientation of the fourth generation's policies.

reigning in the epidemic. If the effectiveness of these measures vanes and the SARS epidemic persists beyond the summer of 2003 or erupts again in the winter, major political repercussions cannot be ruled out. However, if the present measures are successful in containing the epidemic, the Chinese government will hardly face, as some have argued, its "Chernobyl".

Rather, the SARS crisis is likely to imbue some momentum to fundamental trends already present in China's political economy. At first, the successful handling of the crisis will shift the balance of power within the elite. Some Chinese commentators have pointed their fingers at Jiang Zemin, noting that he had supreme power during the months of the initial SARS outbreak, but had chosen to do nothing.[24] Regardless of how Jiang Zemin's role will be judged, the hands of Hu Jintao and Wen Jiabao are being strengthened. Their candor and highly visible management of the SARS epidemic has improved their legitimacy within the party and among the public.

The strengthening of the power base of the two core leaders of the fourth generation will in turn create a window of opportunity for change. Ultimately, Hu Jintao and Wen Jiabao have made a small gamble. They have presented a more humane and amenable face to China's public. Especially now that China's middle classes are disillusioned with how the system handled the epidemic, and foreign investors have lost a degree of confidence in China, there is immense pressure on these two leaders to follow through on their words. To what degree new policy initiatives will emerge is still uncertain. In

---

[24] Bruce Gilley, "SARS Plays into Beijing's Hands," *Asian Wall Street Journal*, May 1, 2003, p. A7.

fact, it is likely that once the SARS crisis passes, China will return to politics as usual. Nonetheless, the shock to China's political and social system created by SARS is liable to cause a reorientation of the fourth generation's policies.

Definitely, there will be stronger emphasis on healthcare and social security reform. The discourse of government will also pay more attention to issues of social justice and inequality. More problematic will be a continuation of the recent trend towards greater government transparency and more open press reporting. Some backtracking in this arena is likely. Perhaps most difficult will be the establishment of a more pronounced culture of governmental accountability, since this could directly hurt the interests of local government officials. Despite these obstacles, the battle against SARS and the handling of its aftermath is about shoring up the credibility of China's party-state. The legitimate rule of Hu Jintao and Wen Jiabao rests on their putting newfound touch of humanity to work. China will remain an authoritarian and repressive state, but it will need to shift its political economy from a raw and brutal form of capitalism to a more humane and compassionate form.

CHRISTOPHER A. MCNALLY

Dr. Christopher A. McNally joined the East-West Center in the year 2000. His research interests focus on the political economy of China's reforms with emphasis on the following subject areas: the political implications of the rise of private firms in China; China's western development strategy; the dynamics of contemporary capitalism in the Asia Pacific and their impact on China; and the implications of China's growing economic power on the East Asian security environment.

Dr. McNally has had research fellowships at the Asia Research Centre, Murdoch University, West Australia and the Institute of Asia Pacific Studies, The Chinese University of Hong Kong, as well as two years of fieldwork under the auspices of the Shanghai Academy of Social Sciences. He received his B.A in Asian Studies from the University of California at Berkeley and his Ph.D. in Political Science from the University of Washington.

He has authored numerous publications including *The Significance of Political Networks in China's Private Sector*, *The Great Western Development Strategy in Sichuan Province*, *Strange Bedfellows: Communist Party Institutions and New Governance Mechanisms in Chinese State Holding Corporations*, and *The Political Dynamics of China's State Sector Reforms*.

Contact details:
Dr. Christopher A. McNally
Research Fellow
Politics, Governance and Security Studies
East-West Center, Hawaii
E-mail: McNallyC@EastWestCenter.org

Section III

Hong Kong

5

The Impact of SARS on Hong Kong Society and Culture: Some Personal Reflections

by *Leo Ou-fan Lee*

To write about SARS in a post-SARS context in Hong Kong runs the risk of sounding rather familiar and dated. Still, I have to fulfill a promise made two months ago to write such an article in English, after I completed a long article in Chinese in early May. The following is not exactly a duplication of that article but both a reiteration of some of my ideas contained therein and some further afterthoughts in a personal vein. My point of departure is the present moment (July 7), a week after the demonstration on July 1 which has triggered perhaps the biggest political crisis since Hong Kong's return to Chinese sovereignty in 1997. The quick succession of these two major crises within a few months has put the increasing polarity between government and society,

> **The Hong Kong government seems to have little patience in learning from the past. Even before the World Health Organization lifted its travel ban, the government had already embarked upon a publicity campaign to attract international attention in order to bring money and investment back to Hong Kong.**

between Tung Chee-hwa's ruling elite and the disfranchised Hong Kong people, in sharp relief. This is unprecedented in Hong Kong's long history. Thus my own reflections on the SAR impact bear a direct imprint of SARS ("Special Autonomous Region") politics: the pun in the nomenclatures is both fortuitous and, in this case, intended.

1.

"Hong Kong was hit hard" — this seems to be a general consensus in the international community. But how hard? How was it compared to Guangdong, Beijing, Taipei, and Singapore? Each place, of course, would claim its rightful share of misfortune. What remains to be seen, however, is how they face the memory of this tortured past and learn some lessons from it. The Hong Kong government seems to have little patience in learning from the past. Even before the World Health Organization lifted its travel ban, the government had already embarked upon a publicity campaign to attract international attention in order to bring money and investment back to Hong Kong. (Although an international commission has been established to look into the structural and operational deficiencies during the SARS era, no one except the government is expecting any significant or unusual findings from its deliberations.) As of this writing, the latest news is that the SAR government plans to stage a number of "spectacles", including a football match starring the world renowned Royal Madrid team with its recently hired English star, David

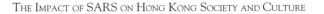

Beckham. There are also reports that former U.S. president Bill Clinton and a few other dignitaries have also been invited to be Hong Kong's "spokesmen." At what exorbitant fees nobody seems to know or care.

I am not surprised by this publicity stunt; the PR campaigns are always a specialty of official Hong Kong culture. Indeed, Hong Kong itself is often seen by outsiders as a "spectacle" — city of glittering skylines and towering skyscrapers in which people are engaged in frenzied commercial activities. Calling itself "Asia's World City," Hong Kong seems rather to fit the category of what the postmodern architect and theorist Rem Koolhaas has called "generic cities" (the other prime candidate is Singapore) — cities which look all alike, with no distinctive individual character except for their mishmash of commodity and tourist attractions. To make up for its lack of interest in any cultural "substance," the SARS government can only attempt to reinvent itself, after SARS, by staging spectacular shows in order to attract more tourists. However, this surface glitter is now enshrouded — or totally eclipsed, according to the foreign press — by the darkening shadows of a gathering storm of popular discontent. The storm finally burst out on July 1 with the march of some half a million people protesting against the government's impending legislation of Article 23 of the Basic Law. The protest sent a clear signal that the majority of the Hong Kong people (nearly 77% according to one poll) have lost faith in their government. Despite the government's attempt at reconciliation by first promising to reconsider three controversial items in the draft of Article 23 and then abruptly announcing the postponement of its final phase of legislation, the people's sentiment is not appeased. Thus, it is now obvious to all parties concerned that the widening gap between government and people is nearly unbridgeable. The SARS episode can now be seen as but the last step in hastening the decline of the SAR government's authority.

The storm finally burst out on July 1 with the march of some half a million people protesting against the government's impending legislation of Article 23 of the Basic Law.

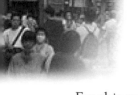

For this writer at least, it confirms once again the typical feature of the government's "managerial" style, namely its excessive reliance on institutional procedures: memorandums, reports, meetings, consultations, etc. *ad nauseam*, before any action can be taken. I have elsewhere called it the manifestation of an "excessive modernity" syndrome. This naïve belief that procedural "rationality" — a vulgarized practical notion derived from Max Weber — seems to have been so deeply ingrained in the minds of Hong Kong bureaucrats that they cannot imagine any alternative way of "doing business." Some critics have faulted British colonialism for this mind-set. But I think the roots go much deeper and wider. It has long been observed that Tung Chee-Hwa's style of leadership is patriarchal and derived from essentially the Confucian tradition. As such it makes interesting comparison with Singapore, where Confucian ethics, also considered a central component of what was once fashionably called "Asian values," has been actively promoted officially. Yet the conduct of the Singaporean government during the SARS campaign, it seems to me, was more creative and flexible. This contrast seems to put Hong Kong in a bad light. On the other hand, the more high-handed measures adopted by the Chinese government under its new leadership are applauded everywhere, despite its initial attempts at covering up. Still, few commentators seem aware that such high-handed measures are only possible within an authoritarian political structure, in which availability of information is still a matter of governmental control. Needless to add, the Taiwan situation was an even worse mess than in Hong Kong, the issue no doubted crowded by the political interests of all the parties. The above comparison seems to be the general consensus among commentators.

To be sure, the style of "procedural" management bears the positive imprint of democratic politics, but its defects are also obvious. For it tends to be bogged down by too many procedural rules and much paperwork and the final decision can only be arrived at slowly, at the end of a long process. This is further complicated by the potential collision between those functionaries who rose from the usual bureaucratic ladder and those who do not have the bureacratic background but are drafted for service by Tung himself. Often the two groups do not see eye to eye. That such a style does not provide an efficient way for conflict resolution goes without saying. In case of internal debate and dissension, the final decision is often delayed and hence "falls a few steps behind." (This has become one of the most commonly used phrases by the Hong Kong press.)

In case of internal debate and dissension, the final decision is often delayed and hence "falls a few steps behind."

The response of the SAR government's medical bureaucracy during the SARS period is a case in point. In the initial period in March, it was taken by surprise and hence unprepared: its operational structures failed to meet the emergency demands created, in particular, by the massive contagion of Amoy Gardens residents. As several public hospitals tried to cope with this unusual attack of an unknown virus on the "front line," the medical support system fell behind, thus causing more anxiety and anger. But the case is more complicated as it involved the precarious linkage between the public hospitals on the one hand and the government's medical administration on the other. From hindsight, both seem to have suffered from a "malaise of modernity," the over-confidence in modern technology and "instrumental rationality."

Hong Kong's public hospitals, such as the Prince Wales or the Princess Margaret, have long prided themselves for being the most "advanced" in their modern facilities and professional staff. Yet they proved to be no match for the SARS virus, which easily infected patients and doctors alike. Apparently something went wrong, aside from the lack of detailed medical information. Probably the earlier cavalier attitude on the part of doctors was a sign of both negligence (in not wearing proper protective gear) and arrogance. For despite rumors of its outbreak in Guangdong, which circulated several weeks beforehand, no one in the hospitals or in the government's health agencies seemed to pay much attention, until it was too late. As a result, they fell several steps behind. This initial ordeal also proved to be a challenge to the hospital staff, from doctors to the cleaning women, who would show exemplary valor and dedication in reestablishing their professionalism. Now that the doctors and nurses who died are made both martyrs and heroes, one still looks back on their spirit of courage and sacrifice with wonder: Why was it that nobody resigned from service, as a host of Taiwanese doctors did? Was it wholly attributable to their professional ethics? Or was there something else to be found in their "collective" character?

If professional ethics governed all doctors, one would have seen a more conjoined effort of all medical staff from both the public and private hospitals.

97

The "professional" behavior of doctors and nurses who sacrificed their lives exemplifies what in popular Cantonese is called the spirit of "*bok-ming*" or "work one's head off." Hardship goes with hard work and indeed spurs hard work.

However, it was mainly the former that bore the brunt of the SARS attack, with little support from the latter. The two kinds of doctors make interesting comparison. The staff at the public hospitals seemed to take for granted their duty of serving the people. This routine professionalism goes with the job. This is especially true with the lower-ranking staff — nurses, cleaning women, etc. — whose dedication to work has won applause from all sectors of the Hong Kong population. But the private doctors who run small clinics are a different matter. Although a few of them volunteered to combat SARS, the majority of them either closed shop or guarded their turf *against* the appeals for help. The government had to negotiate with them for more beds and other facilities. This private sector in my view represents the other side of Hong Kong modernity, as it serves a different clientele of higher-income patients who are more pressed for time and cannot wait in long lines at the public hospitals. The SARS attack has put the chain of horizontal coordination in disarray: sending SARS patients from one hospital to another entails more bureaucratic procedures and perhaps more cumbersome obstacles than can be known from the outside. This in turn creates a further problem of the "chain of command" — whether the government's top bureaucrat in charge of public health could indeed command these various forces. All these issues will presumably be examined by the international review commission (headed, however, by Dr. Yeoh, the minister of public health!), but they are of little relevance to the purpose of this essay.

My concern, however, lies in the realm of the "human spirit". In my view, the "professional" behavior of doctors and nurses who sacrificed their lives exemplifies what in popular Cantonese is called the spirit of "*bok-ming*" or "work one's head off." Hardship goes with hard work and indeed spurs hard work. This popular ethos is part of a legacy from the sixties and earlier, when

Hong Kong was yet to be a fully modernized society. The memory is now recalled with pride and has been re-invoked from time to time, most recently by Anthony Leung, the Finance Secretary, to cheer up the spirit of the populace from their economic doldrums. However, such a traditional work ethic, which may have served to buttress the spirit of doctors and nurses in the hospitals, does not necessarily square with the larger economic trends of the global market. Why is it that the harder one works now, the poorer one gets? This central economic factor has of course become the shared concern of both the government and the people today, but it is seen from different perspectives.

Obviously, the gap between the rich and the poor in Hong Kong has been visibly widened in recent years — so much so that the two have become two totally separate worlds. The poor sector now includes large numbers from the middle-class who lost their fortune from the high-priced housing market during the late 1990s. Its frustrations are directed against Tung Chee-hwa's cabinet, which consisted almost entirely of wealthy businessmen. With their luxurious mansions on the peak (or at least mid-levels) on the Hong Kong island, their brand-name automobiles (the purchase of one such car without paying the anticipated high tax led to the recent scandal involving Anthony Leung), and their generally more cosmopolitan life-style mixing with the equally rich and famous foreign residents and company heads, this small elite group has very little in common with — and has little understanding of — the average people of Hong Kong. Yet they are in a position to dictate Hong Kong's future development, whereas the average man or woman of the streets feels increasingly powerless. The SARS disaster has served to sharpen and exacerbate this division and refocus the frustrations of the latter onto Tung Chee-hwa himself, who had taken command of the SARS management and proved once again incapable of handling the emergency. Since Tung wished also to take the responsibility alone for his failing bureaucrats, he thus became the easy target on which all kinds of popular frustrations have been concentrated.

The poor sector now includes large numbers from the middle-class who lost their fortune from the high-priced housing market during the late 1990s.

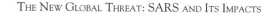

On the other hand, during the worst period of the SARS attack, a common bond was forged between the hospital staff and society at large, due largely to the intervention of the media. Such a bond was used against the government, blaming it for its inability to listen to the collective wisdom of both the specialists in the hospitals and the people. Since the government bureaucracy did not react quickly enough, quite a few nurses and other medical staff appealed directly to the radio-show hosts to complain. The government, therefore, found itself in an increasingly defensive position of having to put up with the barrage of criticisms directed from all corners of Hong Kong society. And given the media domination during the SARS months, the few measures initiated by the government, such as declaring a day of environmental hygiene with high-ranking officials leading the way in cleaning the streets, including the dirty corners at Amoy Gardens, became pathetically ineffectual and roundly ridiculed by the media. Was the government really that bad or did it become merely the most convenient target? One must admit that after the initial disarray and in spite of its internal dissensions, the government bureaucracy finally pulled itself together and managed to cope with the situation more efficiently. But to the populace at large this was still not enough.

The lessons to be drawn from the above are obvious but still beyond the grasp of Tung's cabinet. This was a case not so much of testing bureaucratic efficiency (although it is often seen that way by most people) as of handling emergency. An emergency can either weaken a bureaucracy or strengthen it by virtue of the inspired example of a charismatic leader. It is in this regard that Tung Chee-hwa proved himself to be no Giuliani whatsoever. This comparison may not be fair to Tung or Hong Kong, since in terms of both the nature and the scope of the disaster — of New York after the destruction of World Trade Center and Hong Kong after the SARS attack — the two are not fully comparable. Still, even on the public image front, the shadow of this SARS stigma for Hong Kong will not go away entirely, and more soul-searching as well as more drastic measures must be undertaken by the SAR government

> **A common bond was forged between the hospital staff and society at large, due largely to the intervention of the media.**

before Hong Kong can reassert its former glory. In short, Hong Kong must somehow find ways to re-establish its reputation and "aura" in light of — or in the shade of — increasingly negative predictions about its future.

2.

At the worst time of the SARS epidemic, *Time* magazine chose to publish a special article by a commentator based in Hong Kong predicting its inevitable economic demise as a result of SARS. According to the article's historical "logic," since plagues in history took place more likely in seaports where circulation of people and goods was more frequent, the after-effects always led to their decline and fall. Hong Kong as an international seaport is but the most recent victim, especially in view of its proximity to the epicenter of recent epidemics — southern China, particularly the Pearl River Delta region. If this argument of historical and ecological determinism were to prove valid, no effort from any person or sector in Hong Kong would make any difference in altering Hong Kong's future. Such a "geopolitical" analysis, however, leaves little room for cultural and human considerations. Yet this is precisely what makes Hong Kong at this moment an exciting case for concerned study by both social scientists and humanists, if not by "scientific" soothsayers of doom.

The focus of my reflections — one that is more meaningful to me personally — concerns Hong Kong's society and culture, especially as seen from the inside. If the story about government inefficiency told above has become too familiar, the narrative of how a new popular solidarity was forged during the SARS-infected city whose residents reaffirmed their collective power and voice in the recent protest march is yet to be fully written. I can only piece together a few obvious threads in this human fabric, now woven into an emergent shape of popular sovereignty.

Contrary to the world of instrumental rationality of the Hong Kong governmental bureaucracy — a perfect, though inefficient, model of what socialists would call "*gesselschaft* — I see Hong Kong society largely in human terms as a world of "*gemeinschaft*" whose physical energy and cultural dynamism never cease to amaze me as a half-outsider. However, to reflect upon the SARS impact as a member of this human multitude (for I certainly lived through it myself) also runs the risk of impressionism lacking in objectivity.

Such being the case, I can only claim that what follows represents only my own thoughts and sentiments.

My own "cultural" approach to Hong Kong begins with the world of everyday life. I have written elsewhere about Hong Kong's quotidian culture, a culture that draws its energy from both the popular ethic of hard work ("*bok-ming*") and hard "play" ("*wan,*"always as a verb). To be sure, this description of culture can be applied to most other Asian societies. Still, Hong Kong people pride themselves in the exuberance and even excessiveness of their everyday activities: aside from going to work on the subway or bus in all haste, they would crowd the restaurants and shopping malls everyday with frenzied eating and buying; their activism is especially hectic during weekends and holidays with excursions to scenic sights near or far and frequent tours abroad during the summer season. Media plays a major role in whipping up the popular appetite and sustaining their desire, so that the energy level is maintained at high pitch at all times. For a relatively small but over-crowded city, the range and diversity of cultural rituals and resources — from Cantonese diem sum to Western high tea, from small gatherings of old women at the local MacDonald's to extravagant dinner parties for thousands, not to mention the variety of commodities and goods from everywhere — are immense and ready to be partaken by the activity-driven residents. This familiar picture (which nevertheless provided the key source of inspiration for the beginning scenes of the famous Hollywood science-fiction movie, "Blade Runner") is what makes Hong Kong such a bustling "city of life," Hong Kong's official slogan. For the casual tourist, Hong Kong is also an "empire of signs"; no other city I have visited can remotely compare with the density and omnipresence of advertising: on television and in newspapers (even occupying the full front page), on subway stations and buses and minivans, and on streets and in shopping malls. Needless to add, the visual and noise "pollution" created is equal to, if not greater than, that of any other Asian city.

In my view, the impact of SARS on Hong Kong society has been ambivalent and contradictory, both negative and positive. In the economic sense, of course the toll is heavy: for three months, Hong Kong was a "besieged" city and all activities of consumption seemed to stand still; classes were suspended and people generally stayed at home and did not venture out into their familiar restaurants and malls. The scene of a quiet and withdrawn city is utterly contrary to its character and self-image. Thus one of the SAR government's first post-SARS efforts was to encourage popular consumption, with high

102

This new communal spirit was further promoted by the mass media which for once began to serve a constructive purpose by informing the public not only of the most recent news of the SARS outbreak affecting the housing compounds, but also of the methods of coping with it in everyday living.

officials leading the way of shopping! On the other hand, the silent fear and suffering at home also served to forge a bond out of a sense of common awareness. Here the incident at Amoy Gardens can be cited as an example. The sudden contagion of the SARS virus initially alarmed the residents and made them cantankerous. When the government finally decided to evacuate some residents from the Amoy Gardens to other designated areas for quarantine purposes, the effort met with resistance. (The same happened in Taiwan, on an even larger scale). Yet during the two weeks when they were forced to be together, the residents who normally never bothered to know their neighbors were able to strike up a common chord. So instead of mutual accusations, a spirit of mutual help gained the upper hand and seemed to have extended everywhere. This new communal spirit was further promoted by the mass media which for once began to serve a constructive purpose by informing the public not only of the most recent news of the SARS outbreak affecting the housing compounds, but also of the methods of coping with it in everyday living. In so doing it has created an "imagined community" of people who share the same fate and communal bond. The clarion-calls from media to raise funds to help the hospital staff and their dead met with immediate and unprecedented response. Even the English-language community joined the common cause. For instance, the "Project Shield" campaign launched by the English-language newspaper, *South China Morning Post*, raised millions in a matter of days, with large donations coming from Hong Kong's foreign minorities — Indians, Nepalese, Filipinos, as well as Europeans and Americans — who all consider Hong Kong to be their *home*. This new sense of being "homed" in turn served as an invisible weapon against the "alien" SARS attack, which threatened initially to "un-home" some residents.

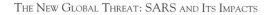
The more effective public medium for this invisible bond was the public radio, which became a ready channel for oral complaints against the government as well as the free exchange of ideas and feelings among listeners. The "hero" on the sound waves was surely Cheng Kinghan (Zheng Jinghan, nicknamed "Taipan Cheng") who assumed the role of a popular commander-in-chief by rebuking high officials who appeared on his show, "Teacup in the Storm," and by rallying support behind the frontline doctors and nurses. (He was, however, forced to take a long vacation under governmental pressure after SARS was over.) Thus media became the true "intermediary" that united different segments of the people and publicized their cause. If, according to some postmodern theorists such as Jean Baudrillard, present reality is being replaced by the "simulacrum" or "virtual reality" of media, the latter in turn brought an unusual "reality" — SARS — to bear on the average Hong Kong citizens and helped them in coping with it more effectively than any bureaucratic measure. (In fact, one of the more effective means used by the government was also to publicize via media, as when some of the officials in charge of hygiene and education appeared in television ads to announce the government policies.)

Thus one local commentator has declared that SARS has in fact helped the Hong Kong people — natives and foreigners alike — find a new collective identity, one that has nothing to do with Tung Chee-Hwa's government. In other words, the recognition of communal power seems to have paved the way for the construction of a new "civil society." Whether or not we can call it a "civil society" in the original sense formulated by Habermas is debatable. But there is no denying the fact that the most active participants in the anti-SARS struggle come from, aside from hospital staff, Hong Kong's non-governmental sectors: the media, university students, religious groups, entertainment industry, even commercial outfits and publicity agencies, as well as residents in housing communities such as the Amoy Gardens — whereas the actors in the political arena (party politicians, legislators, and other local representatives, even the usual anti-government activists) played only a minor role. The imprint of this communal spirit, now celebrated in numerous "heart-to-heart" campaigns and commercials, is visible everywhere and even used by the government to buttress its own reputation. If such indeed is the result, it only goes to show that the ultimate winner in this entire SARS war is not the government but the people. A notable feature of the July 1 demonstrations was the supreme confidence on the part of the marchers, who not only kept up their orderly behavior during the long three-hour wait in Victoria Park before they could throng the streets, but articulated their demands and pleas with visual and verbal flair. Unlike the Tiananmen Square democracy march of students who became increasingly radicalized, the Hong Kong demonstrators kept up the moderate but carnival-like atmosphere while fully aware of the significance of their action. The communal spirit thus also serves to instigate a new social movement which may well enact the age-old tradition of civil disobedience if the government fails in its effort at accommodation.

Several local commentators have called it a new Hong Kong "identity" on the rise — an identity based in communal sharing and forged in a time of adversity, whose contours are neither "national" (as it is not directed against the government in China) nor "provincial" (as it does not have much in common with Guangdong or Shenzhen) but "Hong Kong specific," as it stems from Hong Kong's particular plight in the present. From hindsight, it can be said that the SARS epidemic has crippled the government of the "Special Autonomous Region", but it has also brought about something that makes Hong Kong, as a special city/region, truly "special" (if not autonomous). I should also admit that I am proud to have contributed a small share to Hong Kong culture by doing what I do best professionally — that is, teaching literature. During and after SARS, I have consciously embarked on a personal campaign to write and speak in pubic so as to encourage Hong Kong residents to read more literary classics (such as Albert Camus's famous novel *The Plague*) — if only to give one more source of spiritual comfort and one more incentive for all of us to endure and live on. As to how I read such "classical literature" in the immediate context of a SARS-infected city, the topic belongs to another paper.

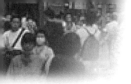

LEO OU-FAN LEE

Dr. Leo Ou-fan Lee is currently P.K. Pao Distinguished Visiting Professor at the Hong Kong University of Science and Technology. He has been professor of Chinese Literature at Harvard since 1994, having taught at several other American universities, including Chicago, Indiana and UCLA. His publications include *Shanghai Modern* in English and a dozen collections of essays in Chinese.

Correspondence to: Prof. Leo Ou-fan Lee, E-mail: hmllee@ust.hk.

6

SARS and the HKSAR Governing Crisis

by *MA NGOK*

The outbreak of Severe Acute Respiratory Syndrome (SARS) in the Hong Kong Special Administrative Region (HKSAR) in March to May 2003 had taken more than 290 lives in Hong Kong, with more than 1,700 infected during that period. The epidemic has also had a huge negative impact on the already ailing Hong Kong economy. More importantly, it has led to lower confidence on the part of the Hong Kong citizens on the government, aggravating the governing crisis. The Hong Kong public was in general not satisfied with the performance of the HKSAR government in its handling of the crisis, the view being that the SAR administration in general, and Chief Executive Tung Chee-hwa in particular, were at least partly to blame for the huge human and economic losses. If there was any blessing in the crisis, it is

Correspondence address: Division of Social Science, Hong Kong University of Science and Technology, Clear Water Bay, Hong Kong. Tel: (+852) 2358-7839, Fax: (852)-2335-0014, E-mail: soma@ust.hk

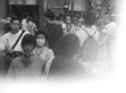

that a new community spirit has arisen, as evidenced by signs of better solidarity, and of a more caring and tolerant society that has resulted.

The Outbreak of the Crisis

The outbreak of the SARS epidemic in Hong Kong could be traced to one patient who was admitted into the Prince of Wales (POW) Hospital on March 4, 2003. At that time, the community (including perhaps the Hong Kong medical community) had little knowledge about SARS or atypical pneumonia (AP). One week later, 18 medical staff who had been in contact with the patient were found to have AP and were hospitalized. By March 13, 33 people in the POW Hospital had fallen sick due to AP, including medical doctors and 17 medical students from The Chinese University of Hong Kong (affiliated to POW). Medical staff at the hospital feared that there could be a major outbreak in the community. However, Secretary for Health, Welfare and Food, Yeoh Eng-kiong insisted on March 17 that the spread was limited to medical staff and relatives of the patients, and there were no signs that the disease was being spread to the community.

The development of events quickly proved Yeoh wrong. In the week after he made the speech, on average 20 patients were hospitalized every day because of AP, many of whom were not medical staff. On March 23, the administration was shocked when it was confirmed that Dr. William Ho, Chief Executive of the Hospital Authority, the public body responsible for managing all public hospitals, had contracted SARS. Ho was infected during his frequent visits to hospitals, showing that the disease was in fact highly contagious. The SAR administration was forced to admit that the SARS virus could be spread to the community quite easily, and more decisive precautionary measures had to be taken.

The outbreak quickly became a hot news topic in both the local and international media. For weeks in Hong Kong, there was almost no other news apart from news related to SARS; even the war in Iraq took a back seat. The World Health Organization (WHO) issued the travel warning to Hong Kong on April 2, and Hong Kong was seen as the origin of the deadly virus by people all over the world. Community panic in Hong Kong reached a climax with the outbreak in Amoy Gardens, a private housing complex of densely-

For weeks in Hong Kong, there was almost no other news apart from news related to SARS; even the war in Iraq took a back seat.

packed high-rise apartments. Starting from late March, it was discovered that more than 100 Amoy Gardens residents had contracted SARS.[1] As most people in Hong Kong lived in similarly dense housing complexes, and the reason of the outbreak was unknown at the time, it led to much fear about the epidemic. The Hong Kong public was so worried that they avoided going out, bringing a huge negative impact on the consumption market.

Starting from April 2003, the SAR government gradually adopted several measures to put things under control. Relatives of patients, or those who had close contacts with patients, were put under home confinement for ten days. Amoy Gardens residents were put in quarantine camps. Schools were suspended for several weeks. Travelers in and out of Hong Kong had to have their body temperature checked to make sure that they did not have SARS symptoms. Since May 2003, the virus seemed to be largely under control, with the number of people infected dropping to single-digit every day. On May 23, the WHO withdrew the travel warning to Hong Kong. On the following day, Hong Kong recorded the first day with no new infected patients. Hong Kong ceased to be an infected area in June. While medical experts warned that there might be another outbreak in winter, the worst time seemed to be over for the HKSAR.

The Economic Impact of SARS

It was believed that four sectors in Hong Kong were affected most by the SARS epidemic: tourism, entertainment, catering and retail sales. Because most people stayed home during the crisis, local retail sales dropped by more

---

[1] Up until late May, more than 300 SARS patients lived in Amoy Gardens, out of a total of about 1,700.

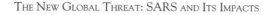

than 50% in the month of April. The catering business was particularly hard hit, leading to closures of as many as 1,000 restaurants and the loss of more than 5,000 jobs. After the WHO issued the travel warning to Hong Kong, tourism was hard hit, with some local travel agencies losing turnover by as much as 90%. Tourism in Hong Kong relied a lot on tourists from mainland China and Taiwan, both of which were having major outbreaks by April. In April 2003 alone, travelers to Hong Kong dropped by 70%. The occupancy rate of major hotels in April was below 10%. Some retail businesses that relied heavily on tourists have also suffered great losses. For example, jewelry retail shops had their turnover reduced by 80–90% during the epidemic.

The epidemic has also hurt normal trade activities. Trade fairs and product exhibitions had to be cancelled, as nobody would come even if they had gone ahead. Because of a general panic of the western world against SARS, Hong Kong business delegations were often refused entry at foreign trade fairs. Jewelry merchants were refused entry at exhibitions in Switzerland, Italy and Las Vegas. Some in the business estimated a loss of 20% in business because of this. As various sectors suffered, unemployment in April rose by 0.2% to 7.8%, with the rate of under-employment rising by 0.3% to 3.2%.

In view of this, the SAR government released a rescue package of 11.8 billion Hong Kong dollars (US$ 1.5 billion)) in late April. The rescue package included reduction of government fees for businesses, reduction of property tax, and rent reduction in government premises. The government offered tax rebates for payers of salary tax, as a gesture to encourage private consumption. The government also put in funds to create 21,500 retraining posts and temporary jobs for workers in affected industries, and for undertaking extra

In view of this, the SAR government released a rescue package of 11.8 billion Hong Kong dollars (US$ 1.5 billion)) in late April. The rescue package included reduction of government fees for businesses, reduction of property tax, and rent reduction in government premises.

Opinion polls showed that most of the Hong Kong citizens were dissatisfied with the performance of the SAR government in handling the crisis.

sanitizing jobs during the epidemic. A special fund of 3.5 billion Hong Kong dollars (US$450 million) was set up to offer loans to the four sectors that were most affected (tourism, catering, retail sales and entertainment).

It is difficult to gauge the exact economic losses caused by SARS to Hong Kong. Some analysts put it as high as $40 billion Hong Kong dollars (US$5 billion).[2] The Asian Development Bank estimated that even if the epidemic was under control by June, it would bring about a loss of 1.2% in GDP growth, with the total loss at three billion US dollars.[3] The economic impacts certainly did not bode well for the popularity of the SAR government. Most of the Hong Kong people, however, were also unhappy with the crisis management ability of the SAR government in handling SARS.

Crisis Management by the HKSAR

On the political front, the SARS crisis has also aggravated the governing crisis of the SAR government. Opinion polls showed that most of the Hong Kong citizens were dissatisfied with the performance of the SAR government in handling the crisis. A survey by the Public Opinion Program of The University of Hong Kong, in April 16–23, showed that only 9% of Hong Kong citizens were satisfied with the performance of the SAR government, reaching an all-time low, while 52% were dissatisfied.[4] Another survey in the same period showed that 58% of the respondents were dissatisfied with the performance of Chief Executive (CE) Tung Chee-hwa in handling the SARS crisis, with only 8.7% satisfied. Sixty-five percent thought he was

---

[2] *Sing Tao Daily News*, May 10, 2003.
[3] *Sing Tao Daily News*, May 10, 2003, p.B15.
[4] www.hkupop.hku.hk/chinese/popexpress/sat_policy/poll/chart/poll7.gif

incompetent as a CE.[5] The public was generally angry at the sluggish response of the government in fighting the SARS outbreak. On May 14, Legislator Albert Chan moved a motion in the Legislative Council, asking Chief Executive Tung to resign, epitomizing societal dissatisfaction. The motion was easily defeated as pro-government members had always been in the majority in the partially democratic Legislative Council. But it was apparent that the SARS epidemic had added to the governing crisis of an already unpopular SAR leadership.[6]

What has gone wrong? The crisis management of SARS revealed several basic problems of the SAR governance. As in similar crises in the past, such as the bird flu crisis in 1997, from the very beginning the SAR government tried to deny there was a crisis, or tried to understate the extent of the problem. When medical doctors at POW Hospital warned openly in mid-March that there might soon be an outbreak in the community, Secretary Yeoh insisted that only medical staff and close relatives of patients were at risk. On March 24, Yeoh admitted that the government had under-estimated the seriousness of the epidemic, and the spread would have been better controlled if the government had imposed preventive measures earlier. This initial attitude hurt the credibility of the government, as the people in Hong Kong believed that the government was not telling the truth and withholding information from the public.

In fact, some felt that the government should have sensed the danger in February, when there was a reported outbreak of hundreds of AP cases in the southern province of Guangdong immediately north of Hong Kong since November 2002. With increasing economic and social integration between Hong Kong and southern China, every week hundreds of thousands of people traveled back and forth between Hong Kong and parts of Guangdong. It could be conceived that the highly contagious disease could easily spread to Hong Kong. However, scenes of Guangdong people scrambling for vinegar[7] in

---

[5] *Apple Daily*, April 22, 2003, p.A1.

[6] For a more complete account of the governing crisis of Hong Kong since 1997, see Lau Siu-kai ed., *The First Tung Chee-hwa Administration: The First Five Years of Hong Kong Special Administrative Region* (Hong Kong: Chinese University Press, 2002).

[7] Some residents in Guangdong believed in a traditional recipe of killing germs by heating vinegar at home, leading to a scramble for vinegar after the outbreak.

The civil servants in Hong Kong favored the rhetoric of "stability", "business as usual", and "orderliness."

February 2003 were dismissed or even ridiculed by Hong Kong residents as irrational or at least unscientific, and the SAR government did not take any special precautionary measures against AP after that. In contrast, the Macau government stepped up precautionary measures, including sanitization of hospitals and public areas, immediately after they obtained the report from Guangdong in February.[8] The result was that Macau had very few reported cases of SARS, while the epidemic ravaged Hong Kong, China and Taiwan.

This inclination to under-emphasize crises had to do with the nature of the administrative state of Hong Kong. For years, Hong Kong has been regarded as a "bureaucratic polity" or an "administrative state" where civil servants dominated policy making, and electoral politicians had little role in making public decisions. As Ku argued, civil servants in Hong Kong favored the rhetoric of "stability", "business as usual", and "orderliness."[9] They had an inherent reluctance to admit crisis, and their training was not well adapted to crisis management. Many felt that the outbreak could have been better controlled if the government had been more alert and warned the public to take appropriate protective measures when SARS first broke out in the POW Hospital.

This aversive attitude to crisis was compounded by two factors. Amidst economic adversity, the SAR government was even more unwilling to reveal bad news, considering that news of an outbreak might bring adverse economic consequences. Secondly, the relevant policy decisions on SARS were mostly made by medical professionals. Secretary Yeoh, Head of Health Department Margaret Chan, and top executives of the Hospital Authority are all medical doctors by training. It was reported that these medical doctors mostly proceeded from a "scientific" point of view, thought the danger and damage of SARS was

---

[8] See *Hong Kong Economic Times*, May 14, 2003, p.A15.
[9] Agnes Ku, "The Public up Against the State: Narrative Cracks and Credibility Crisis in Colonial Hong Kong." *Theory, Culture and Society* 18, 1 (February 2001): 121–144.

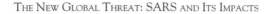

exaggerated by the media, and failed to appreciate the extent of public fear towards the SARS outbreak. For example, Secretary Yeoh had always refused to wear masks in public, since with his medical knowledge he believed that the virus could only be spread by intimate contact, and therefore there was no need to wear masks in normal public occasions such as press conferences. This, however, was contradictory to the government message of asking citizens to wear masks to protect themselves and others. The professional decision-makers also objected to quarantine and home confinement measures at the beginning, because they believed that the scared patients and their relatives would hide from quarantines.[10] To their surprise, in general, Hong Kong people were very cooperative and most did not resist the quarantine measures during the outbreak.

The same situation happened in the case of suspension of schools. On March 25, Education Secretary Arthur Li, himself a medical doctor, said openly that there was no need to suspend schools because "the school is the safest place." However, by that day many primary schools and kindergartens had stopped classes of their own accord, because many parents just would not let their children go to school. While Li might be right in saying that the schools were safer than the community in general, he was rather insensitive to the apprehension of the parents. Two days later, the government was forced to announce the suspension of schools for weeks. It was not until early April, when the community was already in SARS panic, that the government began to understand that it was more important to heed the sentiments and expectations of the public, than to do what is scientifically rational and "correct."

Another major source of public dissatisfaction was that the government seemed to act very slowly in face of the crisis, often lagging behind the course of development of events. The decisions also seemed less decisive when compared to Singapore and Canada. The government agreed to suspend schools only when many schools were forced to suspend classes because of empty classrooms. The measures to rescue the economy were announced weeks after many retail shops and restaurants have closed down. Quarantine measures were imposed on Amoy Gardens Block E only when hundreds from Amoy

---

[10] *Hong Kong Economic Times*, May 7, 2003, p.A3.

Unlike Singapore, Canada or China who assigned or built special hospitals for SARS patients, Hong Kong's SARS patients were initially just admitted to nearby hospitals.

Gardens had fallen sick. At one point the government refused to name the residential blocks that had infected residents, citing privacy concerns. Subsequently, some citizens collected information themselves from hospitals, set up a website and post information on the affected residential blocks. This in the end forced the government to collect the relevant information and announce it later. Most in Hong Kong also failed to understand why the government was slow in enforcing body temperature checks on travelers in and out of Hong Kong. Initially, the government claimed that these measures would slow down customs procedures and cause a jam in border traffic. Then the Shenzhen government managed to set up infrared devices that took only seconds to check body temperature. This was an immediate embarrassment for the SAR government, who quickly installed similar devices days later.

One public institution that took a lot of heat was the Hospital Authority (HA), the statutory body responsible for managing all public hospitals. The HA was first criticized for not fully publicizing the extent of the outbreak in the hospitals and of making inappropriate decisions at the outset of the crisis. Doctors at the POW Hospital complained that when the epidemic first broke out in the hospital, they had suggested to close the hospital to prevent spread to the community, but the request was rejected by HA leaders and government officials.[11]

The HA was also accused of having badly coordinated medical resources during the crisis. Under the HA system, the 42 public hospitals were divided into seven geographical networks, which competed for resources on quasi-market principles. The competition principle was meant to enhance efficiency of service based on managerial principles, but it proved fatal when the government needed to concentrate resources to fight the epidemic. Unlike

---

[11] *Ming Pao*, May 9, 2003.

Singapore, Canada or China who assigned or built special hospitals for SARS patients, Hong Kong's SARS patients were initially just admitted to nearby hospitals. It was reported that at the beginning, different hospital networks refused to let their largest hospital in the network serve as the designated SARS hospital. To balance the interests of different networks, the HA decided to spread the patients evenly to different major hospitals.[12] However, some of these hospitals were not well-equipped to face the crisis, leading to massive contraction of SARS among the medical frontline staff. It was weeks after the POW Hospital outbreak that the government decided to channel all SARS patients to the Princess Margaret Hospital. However, the Princess Margaret Hospital was quickly overloaded when the number of patients hit the hundreds, and many medical staff at the hospital contracted SARS. Then the government decided to move the SARS patients to other hospitals, only to extend a similar problem (though on a smaller scale) to other hospitals.

Since the beginning of the outbreak, there have been repeated complaints from frontline medical staff that they did not have enough protective gears when dealing with patients. There were reports that the HA management in the geographical networks was withholding protective materials to frontline staff, fearing that they would not get the supply later. The inability to protect frontline staff — medical professionals constituting some 20% of the SARS patients — was a major reason for the extent and protracted duration of the outbreak. Legislator Lo Wing-lok, representing the medical professionals' constituency demanded that the HA top management should resign collectively for their failure and mistakes in handling the SARS crisis.[13]

In general, the crisis management experience of the SAR government gave the Hong Kong public the impression that the government was inefficient, badly-coordinated, and non-attentive towards the public's needs and sentiments. The public also doubted the government's sincerity in disclosing full information on the epidemic, as they viewed the government as trying always to withhold information from them. The SARS crisis has severely undermined the confidence of Hong Kong people in the SAR government.

---

[12] *Sing Tao Daily News*, April 27, 2003; *Ming Pao*, May 9, 2003, p.A12.
[13] *Sing Tao Daily News*, April 27, 2003.

The Relationship with China

The relationship with the Central Government was one factor that affected how the SAR government handled SARS. At the beginning of the outbreak in Hong Kong, the most sensitive issue was that the source of the virus was from mainland China. Although the first SARS case was discovered in Guangdong in November 2002, the SAR government was loath to say openly that the virus came from the mainland. For the SAR government, it was just "politically incorrect" to name the mainland as the source of the outbreak, in line with the government's emphasis that Hong Kong's survival is closely tied to economic integration with and support from the mainland.

Before mid-April, PRC officials were still denying that China had a serious SARS problem. Minister of Health Zhang Wenkang claimed that Beijing was a safe place for investors and visitors, and that there was no SARS outbreak in China. The Hong Kong public, however, heard a lot of reports from north of the border that the SARS outbreak in Guangdong was much more serious than reported, and they generally felt that the SARS virus came from the mainland. The acquiescence of the SAR government on the subject was seen by the Hong Kong public as an attempt to cover up for the Central Government, at the expense of Hong Kong's interests. In particular, many felt that the government should give clear instructions whether or not it was safe to go to the mainland, with so many people traveling across the border every day.

The attitude of the Hong Kong public towards the Central Government took a dramatic turn after mid-April. On April 20, the PRC government sacked Minister of Health Zhang and Beijing Mayor Meng Xuelong, for their incompetence in dealing with SARS in Beijing. From then on, the Chinese government took a very positive attitude towards handling of SARS. They admitted that it was a severe problem, released relevant information, and strictly enforced decisive healthcare measures throughout the country. This put immense pressure on the HKSAR government. Most Hong Kong people asked the inevitable question that if the more autocratic Chinese government could dismiss their incompetent officials, then why the "incompetent" SAR officials should not also be held accountable. Media critics and the political opposition questioned if Secretary of Health Yeoh Ein-kiong, whom many considered was doing a poor job of handling the crisis, should not be punished.

117

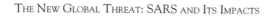

The Central Government was now seen as more open, rational, determined, efficient, and even more accountable to the public than the SAR government.

Worse still, the new attitude of the Central Government led to speculations on the future of Chief Executive Tung. People in Hong Kong felt that if high-level officials in Beijing could be dismissed because of incompetence, the incompetent SAR CE Tung Chee-hwa could also be replaced by the new Chinese leadership. As Tung's strongest support came from former President Jiang Zemin, some hoped the new leadership under Hu Jintao and Wen Jiabao would have a different perspective concerning Hong Kong's affairs. After both Hu and Wen expressed only lukewarm words of support, when asked by reporters about Tung's performance in fighting SARS, rumors spread that the new top leaders were not really happy about Tung. Some rumors went as far as that the Beijing leaders were actually looking for a replacement. This all but aggravated the governing crisis of Tung during the SARS crisis.

Sensing the crisis for the SAR government and Tung himself, the Beijing leaders came out again to openly express support for Tung. In early May, Deputy Premiers Wu Yi and Tang Jiaxun repeatedly offered verbal support for Tung. This temporarily served to quell speculations about Beijing's waning support for Tung Chee-hwa, but did little to solve his impending governing crisis aggravated by SARS.

Societal Responses

If there was any blessing in the SAR epidemic for Hong Kong, it is that the crisis has brought about a renewed sense of community spirit: people displayed greater mutual understanding, rendered more mutual support, and society as a whole has become more caring. This, ironically, happened only after the people had almost lost faith in the SAR government.

At the beginning of the outbreak, the community was in a state of panic. The incident that best illustrated this sentiment took place on April 1. A teenager copied the front-page design of a newspaper on the Internet, made up a "news report" that Hong Kong would be declared an epidemic port on that day, that traveling in and out of Hong Kong would be soon restricted, and circulated it on the web. It was meant to be an April Fool's practical joke, but many people chose to believe it, rushing to the market to pick up food

The different sectors of society soon realized that as the government has failed to provide leadership or timely help, they had to help themselves.

and other daily necessities. Even when the government announced in the afternoon that it was a rumor, that the government had no plans to control traveling in and out of Hong Kong, the scramble to buy goods continued for the whole day. The incident showed that by that time, the Hong Kong public had very little confidence in the words and deeds of the government. Suffering economically and psychologically, the public was in a state of despair, with little confidence in the government's ability to battle the storm.

With the passing of time, however, the different sectors of society soon realized that as the government has failed to provide leadership or timely help, they had to help themselves. More and more groups, business or NGOs, rose to the occasion and joined forces to try to fight the crisis or offer help to those affected. Retailers from the different trades joined hands to offer special discounts to try to lure customers back to their shops. Shop owners formed coalitions to demand rent reduction from landlords. College social work students formed volunteer teams to provide counseling services to victims and those affected by the epidemic. Realizing that the frontline medical staff did not have enough protective gears, political parties and NGOs started donation campaigns to purchase protective masks and gowns to be donated to hospitals. Some felt that the SAR government did not disclose full information about SARS, or was too slow in doing so, so they set up their own websites, did their own information gathering and shared SARS information on the web. Come May, several funds were set up to collect donations to help the victims or their children or frontline medical staff. The funds received active support from the business sector, the government, and the community at large, collecting tens of millions dollars of donations in a matter of weeks.

The Hong Kong community showed special sympathy and support for the frontline medical professionals. From March to May, more than 300 medical staff contracted SARS in the course of their work, and at least seven died subsequently. The Hong Kong people became more appreciative of the

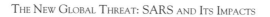

> **The medical workers who gave their lives to save people were deemed community heroes, brave soldiers who died at the battlefront because of inferior weapons and incompetent generals.**

professionalism of the medical staff when they saw TV news reports that medical staff in Taiwan fled from hospitals or resigned from their jobs for fear of contracting SARS. In contrast, medical professionals in Hong Kong did not shirk from their duties; some even volunteered to help the SARS victims. The medical workers who gave their lives to save people were deemed community heroes, brave soldiers who died at the battlefront because of inferior weapons and incompetent generals. The Asian edition of the *Time* magazine dubbed the Hong Kong medical workers "Asian Heroes 2003".[14]

Conclusion

Immediately after the WHO lifted the travel warning to Hong Kong, the SAR government began to work on several fronts for the revival of Hong Kong. The government was planning to hold glamorous international events and large-scale promotion campaigns to regain the confidence of international travelers in Hong Kong. The government also plans to take a more proactive approach in community cleaning, and impose tougher penalties on littering. CE Tung Chee-hwa appointed a committee of international experts, chaired by Secretary Yeoh, to review the whole system of public health.

From the very beginning, the acronym SARS was seen as ominous for the HKSAR. Some said it was the worst crisis Hong Kong has experienced since the Second World War. However, it was also clear that the Hong Kong people emerged from the crisis with a better community spirit and a clearer view of the limitations and strengths of Hong Kong. Would the crisis lead to a

---

[14] *Time*, April 28, 2003.

fundamental resuscitation of SAR governance? Would it lead to a complete overhaul of the current healthcare or hospital system? Will the community be dedicated enough to drastically improve public hygiene, to give the name "the fragrant harbor" its due? Would it lead to a fundamental change of HongKongers' culture, that is, from being a pragmatic and apathetic society, to being a more caring society in which there is greater mutual support and solidarity among people? These are all tough questions for the whole Hong Kong community to answer. The economic impacts can be temporary. If the SARS crisis leads to a fundamental resuscitation of SAR's future, or renewed community spirit in building a post-SARS SAR, the crisis may prove to be a blessing in disguise.

At this moment, there are few positive signs for a fundamental change. "Clean Hong Kong" campaigns have been going on since the 1970s, but public sanitation is still less than desirable. The committee to review the SARS crisis management is chaired by Secretary Yeoh, whom many felt should himself be held accountable for the government's unsatisfactory performance. The review may lead to a re-centralization of power over medical services, not necessarily towards better service or a system more sensitive to people's needs. The crisis, to a certain extent, was rooted in the SAR government's attitude to governance and public opinion. The Tung leadership may be willing to overhaul the medical institutions, but are clearly unprepared to reflect on their philosophy of governance and attitude to public opinion.

MA NGOK

Dr. Ma Ngok obtained his B.S.Sc. and M.Phil degree from The Chinese University of Hong Kong's Department of Journalism and Communication, and Department of Government and Public Administration respectively. He attained his Ph.D. of Political Science from the University of California at Los Angeles. He is currently Assistant Professor in the Division of Social Science, The Hong Kong University of Science and Technology. His research areas include party politics and elections in Hong Kong, comparative politics, political economy and the post-communist transformation in East-Central Europe. He currently focuses on teaching and researching on a wide range of issues concerning post-1997 political development in Hong Kong.

7

The Social Impact of SARS: Sustainable Action for the Rejuvenation of Society

by *Cecilia L.W. Chan*

1. SARS: A New Social Problem

The outbreak of SARS (Severe Acute Respiratory Syndrome) constitutes a new social problem. As well as being an infectious disease, it is also a social affliction that alienates the population, creates isolation, engenders barriers between people, introduces fear to every human encounter, reinforces discrimination and prejudice, removes people's sense of security, and adversely affects community mental health. It has threatened the political, economic, and social stability of Asian cities such as Singapore, Beijing, Taipei, and

Correspondence address: Centre on Behavioral Health, G/F, Pauline Chan Building, 10, Sassoon Road, Hong Kong. Tel: (+852) 2589-0501, Fax: (+852) 2816-6710, E-mail: cecichan@hku.hk

Hong Kong. SARS has had a negative impact on the rate of economic growth, the healthcare system, trade, tourism, and employment: more broadly it has also affected people's sense of global harmony and security, Asian pride and virtually every aspect of daily life.

As of 1 July 2003, a total of 8445 probable SARS cases — 9.6% died, 2.5% still in hospital and 87.9% in recovery — had been reported in more than 30 countries. The WHO issued a global health alert on 13 March after several outbreaks had been reported worldwide. SARS has become a global health issue.

No other virus is similarly threatening. Even the threats of HIV/AIDS, the so-called "mad-cow" disease, hand, foot and mouth disease, and avian flu seem trivial compared with this new and deadly phenomenon. Reports of SARS being transmitted via sitting next to a carrier on an airplane, train, or bus are most alarming. When social contact in public transportations or lifts can be a possible source of infection, simply leaving home to go to work or school becomes a high-risk behavior.

In Hong Kong itself, as of mid June 2003, there had been 1755 SARS cases resulting in 298 deaths. This number is small compared with the 55 new diagnoses of cancer, 20 persons suffering from stroke, and 40 hospital admissions as a result of accidents, injury, and poisoning, which occur each day in Hong Kong. These illnesses and injuries, however, are less worrying because the sick or injured persons will generally not infect their family members when they return home. SARS's unknown etiology, its invisibility, and the high chance of infecting family members remain its most worrying aspects.

2. Hong Kong: The Global Traffic Route

With tens of thousands of passengers per day transiting Hong Kong via airplane, the city has unfortunately become an important site through which the SARS virus is being disseminated worldwide. The epidemic first came to light in November 2002 in Guangdong. However, reports of its prevalence subsided as Guangdong officials exerted pressure on the media.[1] The first index patient,

---

[1] Wang, J.M. and Ji, Z.M., "Control on the media on Guangdong affecting the epidemic of Hong Kong," *Yazhu Zhoukan*, April 28–May 4, pp. 24–29, 2003.

a medical professor from Zhongshan University, went to Hong Kong for treatment on 21 February 2003 and infected a group of people in a hotel in which he stayed for only one day. A few infected guests living on the ninth floor of this hotel became carriers of SARS, passing the virus not only to the Prince of Wales Hospital in Hong Kong but also to Vietnam, Toronto, and Singapore.

As the symptoms of fever, muscle aches, and cough are nonspecific, it is very hard to differentiate SARS infection from the large number of other common viral diseases. Diagnostic delays may therefore contribute to the spread of the epidemic. Key index patients will spread SARS to their family members and fellow hospital patients, and to the healthcare professionals who take care of them. In this way, the first index patient at the Prince of Wales Hospital spread the disease to fellow patients, medical students, and professors looking after him.[2] Unfortunately, the spread then went out of control because the professionals knew very little about the illness.[3]

A 33-year-old index patient with chronic renal failure caught the virus during his visit to the Prince of Wales Hospital. Being a silent super-carrier, he disseminated the virus to residents at Amoy Gardens through his discharges between 14–19 March 2003, while he was staying with his brother who lived in Block E of the development. The inherent nature of the building's architectural design and of its drainage system facilitated further spread of the virus to a large number of residents. As of May 13, 329 residents at Amoy Gardens have been infected.

One Amoy Gardens resident visited his brother in Taiwan, infecting him and also a passenger on a train, who subsequently spread the virus to a large group in Taiwan. An elderly man from mainland China, who had caught the virus from his niece who worked in the Prince of Wales Hospital, returned to Beijing after his visit to Hong Kong. He infected 17 persons on the plane who then carried the virus to Beijing, Inner Mongolia, and other parts of China.

---

[2] Lee, N.; Hui, D.; Wu, A.; Chan, P.; Cameron, P. and Joynt, G.M., *et al.*, "A major outbreak of severe acute respiratory syndrome in Hong Kong," *N. Eng. J. Med.*, April 2003.

[3] Seto, W.H.; Tsang, D.; Yun, R.W.H.; Ching, T.Y.; Ng, T.K.; Ho, M.; Ho, L.M. and Peiris, J.S.M., "Effectiveness of precautions against droplets and contact in prevention of nosocomial transmission of severe acute respiratory syndrome (SARS)," *Lancet* **361**(9368): 1519–1520, 2003.

The unexpected epidemic of SARS in March 2003 has created a worldwide sense of shock and alarm.

This elderly person also went into three hospitals in Beijing and spread the virus to a large group of healthcare professionals. Thus the SARS epidemic spread like a forest fire in Beijing during April 2003.

3. The Impact of SARS

The unexpected epidemic of SARS in March 2003 has created a worldwide sense of shock and alarm. People feel an overwhelming sense of fear, helplessness, anxiety, and even panic, resulting in an unprecedented challenge to health systems, social cohesion, and public order. This chapter will review the negative and positive impacts of the disease on individuals as well as society as a whole. The following Tables (1 and 2) summarize the principal gains and losses of the SARS experience.

The media often focus on the negative impacts of SARS, such as individual losses, with their heart-breaking stories, and the shortfalls of public administration. Such reports may reinforce myths and exaggerate the likelihood of persons catching the virus. On the other hand, there are also positive reports of heroic doctors and nurses, their commitment to caring for their patients, and the sacrifices that they have made. Over and above the individual level, however, there are also substantial consequences at the societal level. Interpersonal interaction, the economic system, environmental harmony, and international relations are all being affected.

3.1 *The Negative Impact of SARS*

The negative impacts can be understood in terms of their influence on the psychological, social, spiritual, and physical condition of individuals as well as on the societal, economic, environmental, and political dimensions of the global system.

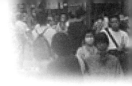

Table 1   Positive and Negative Impacts of SARS on Individuals

Impact of SARS	Negative Impacts	Positive Consequences
Psychological and Emotional	Fear, worry, anxiety and panic	Compassion for the sick and poor
	Blame, meanness and shame	Compassionate loving-kindness
	Guilt of infecting others or being a burden	Resilience and perseverance
	Loss of confidence and feeling confused	Accommodation of differences
	Depression, helplessness and PTSD	Increased emotional strength
Social	Mass hysteria and panic	Social cohesion and cooperation
	Social discrimination against infected persons and their family members	Collective problem solving
	Family conflict and disintegration	Inclusive actions for the disadvantaged
	Social alienation and distancing	Family cohesion and creativity
	Interruption in work or education	Willingness to invest in sustainable development
Spiritual	Loss of meaning, feeling hopeless	Appreciation of life and death
	Emptiness and fear of loss	Re-organization of priorities in life
	Self-pity and Why-Me?	Spiritual reflections, peace of mind
	Blaming God or evil spirits	Active search for meaning
	Denial of self and meaning	Re-affirmation of value, willingness to forgive and let go
	Superstitious practices leading to alienation of groups and individuals	Transformation through pain
Physical	Disease, loss of physical strength	Awareness of importance of personal and public hygiene
	Discomfort due to severe symptoms and side effects of treatment	Rapid technological advancement in treatment and prevention
	Disability especially of long-term lung functions	Learning to take care of the body
	Death	Exercise and physical training

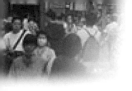

Table 2   Positive and Negative Impacts of SARS on the Economic, Societal, Environmental, and Political Systems of Hong Kong

Impacts	Negative Impacts	Positive Consequences
Economic	Loss of income	Growth in web-based purchasing
	Loss of jobs	New development of eco-industry
	Recession, especially in the service and air transport industries	Improved communication through Internet conferences
	Loss of confidence in investment	Increase in competitiveness due to lowering costs and wage cuts
	Fiscal crisis due to increased public expenditure	Internet business
Societal	Racial and ethnic discrimination	Enhanced sense of community
	Violence, conflict, suicide due to frustration	Improved crisis management
	Greater income disparity	New popular culture and humor
	Growing mistrust among people	Social groups working together
Environmental	Abandoned pets (cats and dogs) on the streets	Investment in environmental hygiene
	Over-packaging of utensils	Public support for improvement in environmental quality
	Mass consumption of bleach and disinfectants	Eco-tourism and development of local cultural tours
Political	Hostility towards authority	International collaboration in the global village
	Disintegration of the healthcare system due to infection of large numbers of medical staff	Demonstration of the importance of transparency of information and public accountability
	Mistrust of government	Enhanced capability of public governance
	Political and social unrest	
	International disputes in trade and travel	

Numerous reports have been made of stress responses and PTSD (post-traumatic stress disorder) after exposure to trauma, mass poisoning, chemical toxin, or mass infection.[4][5][6][7] The most commonly reported psychological effects are anxiety, depression, panic attacks, and PTSD. These emotional symptoms have been found to last much longer than do the physical symptoms and discomfort. Stress and anxiety become more severe when the patient anticipates dying of the disease or of a poisoning episode, or suffering long-term disability.[8]

During the SARS crisis, reports from the mass media have given detailed information on the number of newly infected cases, death rates, geographical distributions, patients' backgrounds, and how they were infected. There have been elaborate reports of the losses people have sustained as a result of SARS (not just deaths but loss of jobs, income, security, sense of joy, and confidence). Dealing with losses is always uncomfortable. These difficult feelings can be expressed negatively as violence and depression.

3.1.1   Fear and Helplessness

Given its highly infectious nature and the level of fatalities involved, the SARS virus has been described as a possible biological weapon. Invisibility

---

[4] Miller, L., "Poisoned minds: toxic trauma, chemical sensitivity, and electrical injury," In Miller, L. ed., *Shocks to the System: Psychotherapy of Traumatic Disability Syndromes*, 1st ed., New York: Norton, (1998), pp. 93–120.

[5] Tarabrina, N.V., Lazebnaia, E.O. and Zelenova, M.E., "Psychological characteristics of post-traumatic stress states in workers dealing with the consequences of the Chernobyl accident," *J. Russian East European Psychol.* **39**(3): 29–42, 2001.

[6] Yokoyama, K., Araki, S., Murata, K., Nishikitani, M., Okumura, T., Ishimatsu, S., Takasu, N. and White, R.F., "Chronic neurobehavioral effects of Tokyo subway sarin poisoning in relation to posttraumatic stress disorder," *Arch. Environ. Health* **53**(4): 249–256, 1998.

[7] Morrow, L.A., Gibson, C., Bagovich, G.R., Stein, L., Condray, R. and Scott, A., " Increased incidence of anxiety and depressive disorders in persons with organic solvent exposure," *Psychosomatic Medicine* **62**(6): 746–750, 2000.

[8] Cwikel, J.G., Abdelgani, A., Goldsmith, J.R., Quastel, M.R. and Yevelson, I.I., "Two-year follow-up study of stress-related disorders among immigrants to Israel from the Chernobyl area," *Environ. Health Persp.* **105**(6): 1545–1550, 1997.

> **Most people who have been interviewed by researchers have developed a highly exaggerated estimate of their own risk of being infected.**

can be horrifying to the public.[9] Such a virus, indistinguishable to the human eye, is just like invisible ink. Once we have touched it, we carry the virus on our hands and deposit it onto all the other materials (files, cups, door bells, lift buttons, telephone receivers, and so on) that we come into contact with. Then, we may touch our mouths or rub our nose and eyes, thus depositing these viruses onto our own bodies. When other people or animals touch the infected objects, they will pick up the virus and become physical carriers. The oral-fecal transmission cycle can only be broken by obsessive hand washing, cleaning with disinfectants, wearing face masks, and avoiding contact with people, especially in enclosed areas such as theatres, restaurants, and karaoke lounges. Such cleaning tasks can be frustrating and tiring.

A number of silent carriers of SARS were admitted to hospitals for broken bones, intestinal bleeding, and other conditions which did not involve fever. These index patients resulted in various outbreaks among hospital staff. More than 370 healthcare professionals have been infected in Hong Kong (to be precise, 379 as at 22 May 2003). Two doctors, a nurse, and a healthcare assistant have already died in the battle against SARS and another 13 remain in critical condition as of the same date.

The public is horrified when it sees nurses and doctors being infected. The common fear expressed is "If doctors and nurses cannot protect themselves from the infection, how can we, as ordinary citizens, succeed in doing so?" Most people who have been interviewed by researchers have developed a highly exaggerated estimate of their own risk of being infected.[10] In a survey

---

[9] Scrignar, C.B., "Invisible trauma: toxic substances, radiation, and pathogenic microorganisms," in Scrignar, C.B. ed., *Post-traumatic Stress Disorder: Diagnosis, Treatment, and Legal Issues*, 3rd ed., New Orleans: Bruno Press, 1996, pp. 69–82.

[10] Department of Community Medicine (2003) Press Conference Materials on the Public Perception and Preventive Measure of Hong Kong Citizens Concerning Atypical (Coronavirus) Pneumonia. 4 April 2003. Hong Kong: Department of Community Medicine, The University of Hong Kong.

conducted by the Department of Community Medicine of the University of Hong Kong during March 2003, about one-third of the respondents (31.4%) estimated that they had a chance of being infected. In reality, there was only 1 in every 4250 persons being infected in Hong Kong. The infected persons were mainly medical staff and people who had had direct contact with super carriers.

A web survey of 1070 students of The University of Hong Kong in April 2003 found a high level of stress (49%) among the respondents. The mental health of the respondents was negatively affected, levels of psychosomatic and stress symptoms were high.[11] Another survey, conducted by the Community Rehabilitation Network of the Society for Rehabilitation, involved 683 chronic patients who took part in telephone interviews in April 2003. Over three-quarters expressed fear of infection and concern about catching SARS and dying of the illness, because of the daily reports of the number of chronic patients fatally infected with SARS.[12] Most of them (64%) were also worried that they would spread the illness to their family members. Women interviewees in particular reported exhaustion due to the level of cleaning tasks required and their concerns about the health of family members.

3.1.2 Collective Grief over Death and Loss

Constant media reporting — as frequent as every half-hour — of the number of infection cases and deaths have placed the population on high alert. People also suffer as a result of hearing about the losses and grief of other families in Hong Kong. Phone-in radio programs broadcast the sad stories of families coping with illness and bereavement. The whole population then vicariously shares the loss and grieving process with these families, as if they were their own brothers. For example, in one family of three, the six-year-old son was in United Christian Hospital (near to Amoy Gardens), his mother was in an acute condition in the ICU (Intensive Care Unit) of Princess Margaret

---

[11] CBH (Centre on Behavioral Health) (2003) Manuscript on the Web Survey on the Psychosocial Distress of SARS. The Centre on Behavioral Health, The University of Hong Kong.

[12] Society for Rehabilitation Survey Report of the Chronic Patients' Views of SARS. 10 May 2003. Hong Kong: Society for Rehabilitation.

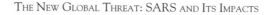

> **Phone-in radio programs broadcast the sad stories of families coping with illness and bereavement. The whole population then vicariously shares the loss and grieving process with these families, as if they were their own brothers.**

Hospital (for infectious diseases), and her husband was in a detention camp for Amoy Gardens residents. The husband called the radio program to share his frustrations about not being allowed to see his wife, who was in a critical condition. He said, "My wife called me and said, I can't breathe, you must come and rescue me." This broadcast resulted in massive public interest in how best to help this family.

After an outbreak of infection amongst mourners at a funeral in Toronto, many people began to refuse to attend the funerals of SARS victims. One husband called a phone-in program and said, "It was only myself and my son carrying a picture of my wife at the funeral. We could not view her body and she was cremated almost immediately. We grieved alone. I feel very guilty not being able to organize a 'proper' funeral for my wife."

Listening to the voices of these grieving individuals every day has prompted the community to go into a period of collective grieving similar to that experienced in New York after September 11. When affected by such a sense of collective loss and traumatization, people can easily develop symptoms of depression and anxiety akin to PTSD. Given the large number of persons being infected and the severity of the consequences, SARS is very similar to a bio-terrorist incident. Anger, panic, irrational thinking about viruses, fear of contagion, attribution of arousal symptoms to infection, and anger with the government are common psychological responses to such traumatic events.[13]

---

[13] Watson, P.J.; Friedman, M.J.; Gibson, L.E.; Ruzek, J.I.; Noris, F.H.; Ritchie, E.C. "Early intervention for trauma related problems," in Ursano, R.J.; Norwood, A.E. (eds.), Trauma and Disaster: Responses and Management. Review of Psychiatry 22(4): 97–124, 2002.

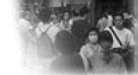

3.1.3 *The Societal Impact*

Feelings of social cohesion and trust, as well as patterns of international exchange, management systems, and public governance, have been shattered. In such extreme cases of panic, people "close up," avoiding social contact and becoming suspicious of others, in order to protect themselves. Schools, hospitals, public gatherings, and even activities in community centers have all been suspended. Frustrations, conflicts, tensions, and stress increase as people do not know what to do.

3.1.3.1 The Loss of Jobs

With this invisible "monster" at large in public places, people have quickly altered their daily routines and leisure activities. Instead of going out to restaurants, they are staying at home. As well as changing their eating habits, families have stopped going to cinemas or air-conditioned shopping malls, preferring instead to have picnics on beaches and in country parks. Spending patterns have changed and the business volume of the service industry has dropped dramatically. Hotels, taxis, and tour groups have lost the majority of their customers, and the employees of affected trades have been forced to take unpaid leave. There is a prevailing sense of helplessness among the population, especially among those whose incomes have been affected.

3.1.3.2 Social and Racial Discrimination

Residents in Amoy Gardens, recovered SARS patients and their family members, and healthcare professionals have felt discriminated against by the public at large. They have shied away from telling others their address or workplace. Similar tensions have been found in Hong Kong, Taipei, Toronto, Singapore, and Beijing.[14]

---

[14] Schlagenhauf, P. and Ashraf, H. "Severe acute respiratory syndrome spreads worldwide," *Lancet*, **361**(9362): 1017, 2003.

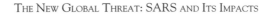

Chinese restaurants round the world are being seen as associated with SARS and people from Hong Kong are regarded as contagious. Home confinement for 10 days has been introduced for Asian students in the UK, Canada, and many other countries.

A series of uncoordinated global movements have arisen in major cities, resulting in discrimination against Chinese people. Airline traffic, trade, and communications have all been affected. Existing anxieties were fueled further by the WHO's travel guidelines advising people against traveling to infected areas. There was a riot by Taiwanese villagers opposed to the treatment of hospital waste materials near their homes. Such episodes of panic can become sources of political and social instability. Residents in Tian Jin broke into a school which had been intended for conversion into a treatment center for SARS patients. Chinese restaurants round the world are being seen as associated with SARS and people from Hong Kong are regarded as contagious. Home confinement for 10 days has been introduced for Asian students in the UK, Canada, and many other countries.

Internationally, a number of trade fairs and major international events have excluded participants from Hong Kong and other infected areas. Many Asian manufacturers lost important opportunities to promote their products at such trade shows. The University of California at Berkeley announced that they would not receive the 500 or more Asian students registered for their 2003 summer school. Similarly, in early May 2003 many US universities asked parents of students from infected areas not to attend their children's graduation ceremonies.

3.1.3.3 Weak Crisis Management

Although the Hong Kong people had been very proud of their hospital systems and the general efficiency of the HKSAR government, they have suddenly come to realize that the public health infrastructure was in fact relatively weak. The public health budget is only one-tenth of the total Hospital Authority budget and none of the 40 publicly funded hospitals contained the well-equipped single person wards necessary for the control of highly infectious diseases like SARS. There were also no changing facilities for healthcare professionals.

This has prompted concern that the SARS outbreak could overwhelm Asian cities' already overcrowded hospitals. Cross-infection in hospitals is also a WHO concern. SARS has created an enormous burden on hospital services. Staff have had to handle a large number of SARS patients without even receiving an adequate supply of protective clothing. Many healthcare professionals have not wanted to return to their homes for fear that they may be infected and in turn will infect their family members. The stresses and worries experienced by their family members have led to the formation of a strong political lobby pressing for better isolation procedures and protection policies for hospital staff.

The government's policies of home confinement, isolation, no hospital visiting, and monitoring of the routes of infection, have been regarded as controversial. The approach taken is a delicate balance between the public interest of disease control and individual freedoms and human rights. The crisis management capacity of the government and the credibility of political leaders have been seriously challenged.

3.1.3.4 Hostility Towards Political Leaders and the Hong Kong Authority

The frustration of knowing so little about the virus, its prevention, treatment, and spread, has been expressed as anger towards the government and authority figures. When microbiology experts informed the community that SARS was likely to become a unique indigenous disease that would stay with us over the long-term, the public directed its anger towards Mr. C.H. Tung, the Chief Executive of Hong Kong. Mr. Tung's popularity fell below 40 points to reach a historical low. Previously pro-government organizations and business groups have become more vocal and more ready to express their grievances or discontent in public. On 14 May 2003, a motion debate was raised in the Legislative Council to invite the Chief Executive to step down.

Similar political tension has emerged in Beijing and Taipei. Political leaders have apologized and incompetent officials have stepped down. The control

A group of professors from The University of Hong Kong started the "We Are with You" (WAY) Movement.

of SARS has turned into a battlefield on which political groups and international bodies have begun to compete for resources, control, and power. The political lobbying of the WHO to remove Toronto and Hong Kong from its travel advisory by the respective governments is a good showcase of international politics at work.

4. The Positive Impact of SARS

Despite the losses due to SARS, its actual impact on individuals and communities has been quite mixed. There are noticeable negative consequences but there are also significant gains. If the population will allow itself to think deeply and reflect on the situation, we can generate meaning out of this traumatic event. Just as there have been both positive and negative impacts from other tragic events like September 11, the same can be true for SARS.

4.1 Gains through SARS

SARS can be turned into a source of positive energy for change, creativity, and innovation. The feelings of shock and loss can become the catalysts for individuals to develop a stronger emotional capacity for change and problem-solving. Those with the ability to reflect on and reconstruct meaning can usually cope more effectively with stress and trauma.[15] These individuals may grow spiritually and be transformed by their experience of trauma or loss.[16]

---

[15] Neimeyer, R.A. ed. *Meaning Reconstruction and the Experience of Loss* (Washington: APA, 2001).

[16] Calhoun, L.G. and Tedeschi, R.G. "Posttraumatic growth: the positive lessons of loss," in Neimeyer, R.A. ed. *Meaning Reconstruction and the Experience of Loss* (Washington: APA, 2001), pp. 157–172.

The WAY produced a new definition of SARS as: Sacrifice, Appreciation, Reflection, and Support. The objective was to promote a sense of empowerment among the population so that people recognized what they could do to help themselves and others.

On April 1, 2003, when there was an outbreak of mass hysteria and people rushed to Hong Kong supermarkets to stockpile food, a group of professors from The University of Hong Kong started the "We Are with You" (WAY) Movement which promoted a "New Definition of SARS." The medical faculties in universities became the trustees of life, of standards, and of academic freedom. The community developed high expectations of universities, seeking academic and research leadership to help Hong Kong move out of the SARS chaos.

The WAY produced a new definition of SARS as: Sacrifice, Appreciation, Reflection, and Support. The objective was to promote a sense of empowerment among the population so that people recognized what they could do to help themselves and others. This SARS was defined as follows:-

Sacrifice: Giving up selfish acts but remaining willing to make sacrifices for the public interest and collective well-being.

Appreciate: Appreciating our strength, the devotion of our professional teams, our family members, and life itself. Adopting an appreciative attitude instead of being mean and discriminatory.

Reflection: Reflection can introduce new learning and meaning. We feel better if there is new wisdom that we can develop through our suffering.

Support: Support for people in need can be a very effective strategy for making new meaning. Care for the disadvantaged can help us grow spiritually and emotionally.

4.1.1 *Turning Curses into Blessings*

If we can develop meaning and consolidate the life lessons of traumatic experiences of loss and pain, we may feel better about having endured the suffering. The meaning reconstruction and meaning making processes are crucial sources of strength helping individuals to cope with their difficulties.[17] Resilience emerges through commitment to a vision, passion for change, faith in perseverance, and trust in a better future. This is evident from a number of studies of post-traumatic growth.

Based on the "Main Findings of an Investigation into the Outbreak of Severe Acute Respiratory Syndrome at Amoy Gardens," a series of recommendations were made on April 17, 2003 and actions taken to educate the public. The aim was to promote community awareness of factors relevant to reducing routes of contamination in the home, such as keeping the U-trap filled with water, employing pest control so as to reduce environmental contamination, keeping the sewage system in good repair and paying attention to the width of the light well in future building regulations so as to avoid the "chimney effect" of contaminated droplets traveling up multi-storey buildings.

On a personal level, we can certainly learn from patients and healthcare professionals. A 16-year-old adolescent was discharged from hospital after surviving SARS but had lost both parents over two days. He said that despite being sad, he was still going to live positively because he had been deeply touched by the devotion and commitment of the healthcare professionals during his hospitalization.

A discharged SARS patient who is also a University of Hong Kong research student shared her notes on her path to recovery with others soon after her discharge from hospital. She had learnt a lot about breathing techniques and physical exercises, as well as gathering information on the use of tonics, herbal medicine, and imagery, during her recovery. Doctors and nurses who have had the experience of being infected have also found the experience valuable as they were able to develop a better understanding of what it is like to be a patient.[18]

---

[17] Chan, C. and Chan, E.K.L. "Enhancing resilience and family health in an Asian context. Special issue of Asian families in crisis: resilience, choices and self-determination," *Asia Pacific J. Soc. Work* **11**: 5–17, 2001.

[18] Ho, W. "Guideline on management of severe acute respiratory syndrome (SARS)," *Lancet*, **361**(9366): 1313–1315, 2003.

Doctors and nurses who have had the experience of being infected have also found the experience valuable as they were able to develop a better understanding of what it is like to be a patient.

4.2 Social Cohesion and the Establishment of Social Infrastructures

The SARS outbreak provides society with an opportunity to become more cohesive. Political parties are willing to work together in confronting the challenges raised by the deadly virus. Songs, books, TV documentaries, radio programs, newspaper columns, CDs, and many other products have been published. Family doctors have formed themselves into district networks to work in old age homes and schools. Psychologists and NGOs have produced community education booklets and CDs to help patients and the community in general overcome their panic and fear.

Individuals and organizations have responded very quickly to the challenge of supporting community education campaigns, fundraising and changing hygiene habits. NGOs have set up hotlines and emergency services, and mobilizing volunteers to distribute facemasks and disinfectants as well as helping underprivileged people to clean up their homes. A group of artists and pop singers produced a song "We Shall Overcome" to boost the morale of the people and to show their appreciation for healthcare professionals.

On April 30, 2003 four senior female government officials initiated an education trust for children who had lost their parents to SARS. They raised US$3 million in less than two weeks. A group of corporations and conscientious community leaders started another fund to help infected patients and their families. They raised more than US$2 million in one day for disbursement by the Social Welfare Department. The ELITE action raised funds for the Hospital Authority and their staff who had been hardest hit by the epidemic. The NGOs and universities initiated hotline services and reached out to the community to help the most underprivileged groups. The

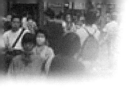

"Fear-buster" movement also pulled together a large group of expatriates to work together to promote Hong Kong locally and internationally. Medical doctors operating in the private market were willing to provide free consultations to chronic patients under the auspices of the Hospital Authority. Individuals, groups, and organizations contributed towards the cause in terms of finances, time, and expertise to help Hong Kong overcome this crisis.

4.2.1 Collective Efforts to Rescue the Service Industries

Seeing the downturn in business among restaurants, cinemas, taxis, air travel, hotels, department stores, and shops, a group of volunteers encouraged Hong Kong residents to leave their homes and spend money. The government introduced tax rebates and other fiscal measures to help the trades most severely affected by SARS. Grassroots projects encouraged citizens to spend US$12 on taxis per week, to go out and eat, to spend money on local tours, and to stay in local hotels. Since the Easter holidays, tour guides previously serving overseas and mainland Chinese visitors, have begun to serve local customers. New routes for local Hong Kong tours have been developed. These local tours have cultivated a sense of pride amongst citizens and developed a new knowledge of local history. Participants have suddenly realized that there are many impressive tourist spots in Hong Kong that they had not previously known about. Standards of service and hygiene in restaurants and food stalls have also improved dramatically.

4.2.2 Physical Infrastructure and Environmental Management

Hong Kong has the world's highest population density with 6411 persons per square kilometer. The localities and districts with the highest number of infected cases have been found to have a much higher population density. For example, Kwun Tong, where Amoy Gardens is situated, has a density of 49861 persons per square kilometer, Wong Tai Sin 47810 persons, Kwai Ching 21578 persons, and Shatin 9157 persons per square kilometer. Our pride in our capacity to locate a large population in cement apartment blocks has been shattered.

In an attempt to learn from the outbreak at Amoy Gardens, which affected more than 350 residents and involved the loss of many lives, architects, planners, and engineers are now trying to establish healthy building guidelines and benchmarking standards for previously neglected areas such as ventilation, open space, hygiene, space between buildings, drainage systems, size of light wells, and preventive management. This crisis can be turned into an active search for indicators and health standards appropriate to a sustainable urban environment.

4.2.3 Technological Advancements

Engineers and architects have begun to contribute to the benchmarking of hygienic buildings. Medical doctors and scientists have been improving treatment and prevention protocols for SARS patients. New markets for drugs and herbal medicines have been developed as people are willing to invest in illness prevention. There has been an increase in the use of communications technology such as tele-conferencing, web teaching, and web selling marketing as a result of SARS, since people have spent more time at home. The daily publicity on the gene mapping of the virus, the size of the air filters required on airplanes to filter it out, the appropriate level of dilution of bleach as a disinfectant, and the infra-red measurement of body temperature have promoted an increase in the public's scientific knowledge and understanding of the latest technologies that can be adopted for infection control. New insights and good practice have been developed and shared to prevent further spread in hospitals.[19] A list of these innovations can be found in Table 3.

4.2.4 Political cohesion and transparency

A number of impressive actions have demonstrated effective governance as a direct result of SARS. For example, mainland China has built a 1000-bed

---

[19] Twu, S.J.; Chen, T.J.; Chen, C.J.; Olsen, S.J.; Lee, L.T.; Fisk, T. et al "Control measures for severe acute respiratory syndrome (SARS) in Taiwan. Emerg Infect Dis [serial online] June, 2003. Available from: URL: http://www.cdc.gov/ncidod/EID/vol9no6/03-0283.htm"

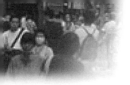

hospital for the treatment of SARS patients and in eight days deployed 1000 army medical staff in Shanghai to work in it.[20] There have also been dramatic improvements in the transparency of reporting of the number of infected persons, enhanced political accountability, and greater collaboration with international organizations such as the WHO.

Despite public complaints about the length of time the government took to make the decision to isolate suspected carriers to curb the infection, the people of Hong Kong can be proud of the exceedingly efficient professional teams involved in the search for solutions in treatment and prevention. The highly transparent political and administrative infrastructures have served as a very good example for our neighboring cities. In any public health decision-making process, there will inevitably be tensions between public interests of infection control (adoption of high-handed, top-down decisions about isolation, confinement, and restrictions on population movement, all of which may contravene the will of the people) versus respect for individual freedom. The necessary precautions must be taken to minimize harm and inconvenience to the population. Hong Kong has tried very hard to strike the delicate balance between these conflicting expectations of individual verus public interests. Awareness of the importance of contingency planning and crisis management has risen. Valuable lessons can be learnt through the process of battling SARS. Table 3 is a checklist of what society can do in terms of sustainable actions over the longer term.

5 Conclusion

The SARS epidemic has hit the world hard. As well as being a physical health hazard, the outbreak has also caused psychosocial and politicoeconomic trauma. Thus, viewing SARS as a social as well as a medical problem can help us to understand and manage the situation better. Learning from the experience of the United States after September 11, we too in Asia can convert this curse into a blessing. By working together, we can mobilize new technology

---

[20] Ashraf, H. China finally throws full weight behind efforts to contain SARS, *Lancet*, **361**(9367): 1439.

and creativity in learning and growing from this experience. We can turn Severe Acute Respiratory Syndrome into Sustainable Action for the Rejuvenation of Society. The SARS epidemic can facilitate spiritual growth in terms of appreciating life and death on an individual level. The external conflict caused by the deadly virus can also lead to internal cohesion among the people of Asian cities. This challenge is a test of the sociopolitical crisis management capability of the affected area. The fear of death has given rise to technological innovation and quantum leaps in scientific and medical research. Although the virus may be indigenous to Asia, we can choose to see it as a curse that is actually a blessing in disguise.

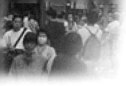

Table 3 Sustainable Actions for the Rejuvenation of Society after SARS

Sustainable Action	Examples
Individual Level	- Enhanced public hygiene standards, public commitment to keeping the city clean, active involvement in cleaning of schools, community, homes, and public places - Health responsibility, wearing masks in case of flu, not going to work or school when sick - Healthy lifestyle; exercise and good mental health - Appreciation and acceptance of the vulnerability of life and death
Family/Neighborhood	- High health standards, investment in public drainage and the communal environment - Taking good care of sick persons at home - Participation in building management, effective refuse collection; learning of bleaching and disinfectant methods; - Encouragement of outdoor activities, increase in public open space
Public Place/Environment	- Frequent disinfecting procedures in public places (schools, shops, office, factories, etc.) - Effective public toilets and cleaning procedures - Clean food processing procedures in restaurants and eating places - Maintenance of high standards in hotels, swimming pools, cinemas, theatres, and shopping malls - Protection of the environment
Health Care/Hospitals	- Investment in public health and disease prevention - Improvement in hospital ventilation, natural lighting and sufficient space to isolate infectious patients to avoid cross-infection - Improvement in reporting systems, reduction in patient concentration, review of medical procedures to enhance protection for professionals
Housing/Architectural Design	- Creation of street canyons to allow effective ventilation and air circulation - Benchmarking of hygienic buildings; improved standards to allow for bigger light wells, improved design to prevent spreading of diseases by better drainage, sewage, and air circulation
Transportation/Technology/Population Movement	- Facilities to prevent infected persons from coming in or moving out of the territory - Effective ventilation in airplanes and other public transport vehicles - Enhanced port health control via UV light and disinfectant; infra-red thermography system

CECILIA L.W. CHAN

Dr. Cecilia Chan is Professor at the Department of Social Work and Social Administration, and Director of the Centre on Behavioural Health of The University of Hong Kong. Prof. Chan is a pioneer in emotions and health. She started a new definition of SARS (Sacrifice, Appreciation, Reflection, Support) under the HKU, and the "We are with You Movement" soon after the outbreak of SARS in Hong Kong. She is a Member of the Society for the Promotion of Hospice Care; and Founder of the CancerLink, Community Support and Information Service, the Hong Kong Cancer Fund. She also contributed to the founding of the Cancer Counseling & Support Service, Queen Mary Hospital, the Cancer Patients' Resource Centre of Queen Elizabeth Hospital, Tuen Mun Hospital and Pamela Youde Eastern Nethersole Hospital. She is a Member of the International Workgroup on Loss, Grief and Bereavement (IWG).

Prof. Chan was Speaker of the 2002 Eileen Younghusband Lecture, International Association of Schools of Social work (IASSW) at the Bi-Annual Conference, France, and Speaker of the 2001 Walter Friedlander Lecture, School of Social Welfare, University of California Berkeley. She was awarded the Hong Kong Baha'i Award For Service to Humanity in 1999; and the Outstanding Social Workers Award in 1994.

Selected Publications

Ran, M.S.; Chan, C.L.W.; Xiang, M.Z. and Wu, Q.H., "Suicide attempts among patients with psychosis in a Chinese rural community," *Acta Psychiatr Scand*, **107**: 430–435, 2003.

Ho, Samuel M.Y.; Ho, Judy; W.C., Chan, Cecilia L.W.; Kwan, Kedo and Tsui, Yenny K.Y., "Decisional consideration of hereditary colon cancer genetic test results among Hong Kong Chinese adults," *Cancer Epidemiol. Biomarkers Prev.* **12**: 426–432, 2003.

Ran, Mao-Sheng; Leff, Julian; Hou, Zai-jin; Xiang, Meng-ze and Chan, Cecilia Lai-Wan, "The characteristics of expressed emotion among relatives of patient with schizophrenia in Chengdu, China," *Culture, Med. Psychiatry.* **27**: 95–106, 2003.

Ho, Smuel M.Y.; Wong, K.F.; Chan, Cecilia L.W.; Watson, Maggie and Tsui, Yenny K.Y., "Psychometric properties of the Chinese version of the mini-mental adjustment to cancer (mini-MAC) Scale," *Psycho-Oncology*, 2003.

Wong, D.F.K.; Chan, C.L.W.; Law, C.K. and Au, T.Y.W., "Medical social services in accident and emergency departments of hospitals in Hong Kong: Their utilization patterns, functions, and outcomes," *Asia Pacific J. Soc. Work* **12**(2): 8–24, 2002.

Chan, Cecilia L.W.; Yip, Paul S.F.; Ng, Ernest H.Y.; Ho, P.C. and Chan, Celia H.Y., "Gender selection in China: Its meanings and implications," *J. Assisted Reprod. Genetics* **19**(9): 426–430, 2002.

Chan, Cecilia L.W.; Chan, Yu and Lou, Vivien W.Q., "Evaluating an empowerment group for divorced Chinese women in Hong Kong," *Res. Soc. Work Prac.* **12**(4): 558–569, 2002.

Cheung, Grace and Chan, Cecilia, "The Satir model and cultural sensitivity: A Hong Kong reflection," *Contemp. Family Ther.: An Inter. J.* **24**(1): 199–215, 2002.

Ho, Samuel M.Y.; Chow, Amy Y.M.; Chan, Cecilia L.W. and Tsui, Yenny K.Y., "The assessment of grief among Hong Kong Chinese: A preliminary report," *Death Studies*, **26**: 91–98, 2002.

Chan, Cecilia; Ho, Petula S.Y. and Chow, Esther, "A body-mind-spirit model in health: An eastern approach," *Soc. Work Health Care* **34**(3/4): 261–282, 2001.

Wong, TW; Chung, M; Chan, Cecilia, "A survey of medical social services in local Accident and Emergency departments," *Hong Kong J. Emergency Med.*, pp. 135–139, 2001.

Chan, Cecilia and E.K.L. Chan, "Enhancing resilience and family health in asian context," Special Issue of Asian Families in Crisis: Resilience, Choices and Self-Determination, *Asia Pacific J. Soc. Work* **11**: 5–17, 2001.

Ran, Maosheng; Xiang, Mengze; Huang, Mingsheng; Shen, Youhe; Ke, Liantin; Li, Sigan; Lou, Zhongren; Chen, Liwun and Wan, Wun, "A control study of psychoeducational family intervention for relatives of schizophrenics in a Chinese rural community." *Chinese J. Psychiatry*, **34**(2): 98–101, 2001. (in Chinese)

Fielding, Richard and Chan, Cecilia (eds.) *Psychosocial and Palliative Care in Hong Kong: The First Decade.* (Hong Kong: the Hong Kong University Press, 2000).

8

Catching SARS in the HKSAR: Fallout on Economy and Community

by *Yun-Wing Sung*
Fanny M. Cheung

Traditionally, south China has been one of the hotbeds of new viruses. Due to its excellent international links, Hong Kong has been the springboard of these new viruses to the world. In 1968, the Hong Kong Flu, which most likely originated in south China, spread from Hong Kong to the rest of the world, causing 700,000 international deaths between 1968 and 1969. An epidemic from the Avian Flu ("Bird Flu") in 1997, which was transmitted through chickens imported from south China, was only averted after the Hong Kong government ordered the slaughter of millions of chickens. The global outbreak of Severe Acute Respiratory Syndrome (SARS) started in south China in November 2002, and then spread via Hong Kong to Vietnam, Singapore, Canada, and other countries in February 2003. Global travel has accelerated the spread of the disease to other countries. In March 2003, the World Health Organization (WHO) issued a global alert on the outbreak of SARS.

Hong Kong reverted to China in 1997 and was renamed the HKSAR (Hong Kong Special Administrative Region). Despite the political change, Hong Kong remains China's window to the world, in trade, in investment, as well as in transmission of new viruses. The impact of globalization has accentuated the interconnectedness of the global community. "Hong Kong Flu" is regarded as a misnomer in Hong Kong as the virus most likely originated elsewhere. Likewise, the HKSAR Government prefers to use the term "Atypical Pneumonia" rather than SARS as the name bears an unfortunate resemblance to HKSAR. In the short space of 35 years, Hong Kong has the misfortune of being closely associated with two pandemics or near-pandemics.

Like the Hong Kong Flu, SARS was transmitted from south China via Hong Kong to other parts of the world. Despite the worldwide alert and scare, the international fatality rate of SARS so far has been much lower than that of the Hong Kong Flu. The higher infection rate among frontline health workers, on the other hand, makes SARS more debilitating and demoralizing. Compared with the Hong Kong Flu, SARS may be less contagious in the sense that the virus is unlikely to be airborne: SARS can only be transmitted through close contact. This means that SARS can be prevented when protective measures are used and the rest of the world can contain the disease by strict quarantine.

Quarantine measures have made SARS much more pernicious for Hong Kong's economy than the Hong Kong Flu. In early April, WHO issued a travel advisory for travelers to consider postponing all but essential travel to Hong Kong and Guangdong province, China. The travel advisory was lifted in late May. As Hong Kong is an international service hub, its economy would be strangled by prolonged quarantine. Unlike the Hong Kong Flu, the uncertainties about SARS and its economic fallout snowballed into a community trauma. In the 104 days that SARS struck Hong Kong (from early March till 23 June, when Hong Kong was removed from the list of areas with local SARS transmission by the WHO), a total of 1,755 people were infected, including 386 medical workers. Fatalities stood at 296, including 8 medical workers. An estimated 13,300 jobs were lost and 4,000 businesses folded. Up to a million tourists stayed away and 13,783 flights were cancelled

The prospect of modest growth in 2003 was dashed by SARS. In late May, the government revised the 2003 forecast down to 1.5 percent.

(*South China Morning Post*, 24 June 2003). Both the rate of infection (as a proportion of the population) and the fatality rate were the highest in the world.

In this article, we highlight the fallout of SARS on Hong Kong's economy and community, and their interconnectedness. We also discuss the opportunities and lessons gained from the crisis.

Fallout on the Economy

Though the Hong Kong economy has been in crisis since the Asian Financial Crisis of 1997, the Hong Kong economy displayed strong growth momentum in the immediate pre-SARS period. Real GDP (gross domestic product) grew by 5.1 percent in the fourth quarter of 2002, and by 4.5 percent in the first quarter of 2003. While the spread of SARS has hurt the economy starting mid-March, growth for the first quarter was still healthy. The growth was led by exports of goods and services, reflecting the pivotal role of Hong Kong in China's trade and investment. In the fourth quarter of 2002 and the first quarter of 2003, exports of goods grew respectively by 18.4 percent and 19.1 percent, while exports of services grew respectively by 18.1 percent and 12.2 percent. Due to the impending war in the Middle East and the mixed performance of the US and EU economies, growth was expected to slow down after the first quarter, and the pre-SARS official forecast of economic growth for 2003 was 3 percent, which was not bad given the uncertain global economy. However, the prospect of modest growth in 2003 was dashed by SARS. In late May, the government revised the 2003 forecast down to 1.5 percent (*South China Morning Post*, 31 May 2003). ING Financial Markets has also revised the 2003 forecast to 1.5 percent (*Hong Kong Commercial Daily*, 27 June 2003).

SARS has also exacerbated Hong Kong's deflation due to the fall in spending by tourists and local residents. Retailers have aggressively cut prices to boost sales. The Consumer Price Index (CPI) fell by 2.5 percent in May 2003 from a year earlier, distinctly larger than the 1.8 percent in April 2003. The government revised the pre-SARS forecast of 2003 deflation from 1.5 percent to 2.5 percent. In a nutshell, Hong Kong will have lethargic growth accompanied by high unemployment and a continuation of the deflation which started in October 1998 due to a weak economy.

Though Hong Kong, Beijing and Taiwan were removed from WHO's list of infected areas in rapid succession in late June and early July, there is still considerable uncertainty in the pace of economic recovery. The adverse effect on the economy will linger for half a year or more. It will take up to a year to convince tourists, especially leisure tourists, that Hong Kong is really safe.

The impact of SARS on the Hong Kong economy is large because Hong Kong is an international service hub. Services require close person-to-person contacts, unlike manufacturing, where products can be delivered to customers overseas without intimate contacts. The impact of SARS is particularly severe on tourism, catering, retail sales, and the entertainment sector.

Despite the severe economic fallout, the worst is clearly over by June 2003. The hard hit tourist industry has shown strong signs of recovery. The occupancy rate of hotels in Hong Kong fell to a mere 20 percent in April and May, but rebounded to nearly 40 percent in June (*Hong Kong Economic Times*, 23 June 2003). Passenger traffic on the Cathay Pacific, Hong Kong's dominant airline, fell from the pre-SARS level of 33,000 a day to around 4,000 a day in April and May, but rebounded to 11,000 a day in mid-June (*Ming Pao*, 18 June 2003). Both Cathay Pacific and Dragonair plan to resume all flights by September. However, the recovery in leisure tourism will be very gradual. According to the Tourism Board, tourist arrivals will be back to 70 percent of the normal level in March 2004, and the full recovery of tourism will take a year (*Hong Kong Economic Journal*, 24 June 2003). In 2003, the decrease in GDP due to the fall in tourist expenditure is likely to be close to one percent.

The impact of SARS on the Hong Kong economy is large because Hong Kong is an international service hub.

> ## The rate of unemployment, which was at 7.8 percent for the months of February through April, rose to 8.3 percent for the months of March through May, setting a record since 1975.

Local spending has also dropped drastically since the SARS outbreak. The Index of Consumer Confidence in April 2003 has dropped to 55.0 compared with that of 70.0 in December 2002; the Indices of Consumer Sentiment of the corresponding periods are 57.4 and 72.9, respectively. These indices were the lowest since the September 11 terrorist attacks in 2001.[1] The spending by local residents on catering and shopping has started to revive since the middle of May, as Hong Kong made good progress in disease control. The Index of Consumer Confidence returned to 73.2, and the Index of Consumer Sentiment returned to 74.3 at the end of May, after the lifting of the WHO travel advisory.[2] Consumption of local residents will be likely to be close to normal in June. The fall in consumption is likely to trim GDP growth by 0.8 percent.[3] In late May, the government revised the 2003 forecast of growth of private consumption expenditure from no growth to a decrease of 3 percent.

Besides tourism and retailing, SARS has an adverse impact on the already very weak property market. In the 100 days that SARS struck Hong Kong, turnover in the property market fell to $22 billion from $33 billion a year earlier (*Apple Daily*, 24 June 2003). Though there was a marked increase in turnover in late June as the WHO declared Hong Kong SARS-free, property prices are expected to remain weak with chronic over supply. The rate of unemployment, which was at 7.8 percent for the months of February through April, rose to 8.3 percent for the months of March through May, setting a record since 1975. The figures imply that the unemployment rate for the

---

[1] *"Report on the April 2003 Survey of the Public's Assessment of Hong Kong's Economy"*, Department of Economics, The Chinese University of Hong Kong.

[2] *"Report on the May 2003 Survey of the Public's Assessment of Hong Kong's Economy"*, Department of Economics, The Chinese University of Hong Kong.

[3] "The Hong Kong Economy Facing SARS", *Economic Review*, Bank of China Economics & Planning Department (http://www.bochk.com), April, 2003.

single month of May was around 9 percent. As around 100,000 secondary school and university graduates are expected to enter the labor market in the summer, the unemployment rate is expected to hover around 9 percent or more till September.

SARS would exacerbate Hong Kong's burgeoning fiscal deficit. The government has announced in April a package totaling $11.8 billion, including increased expenditure on health and relief measures. Around $3 billion would be expenditure for medical research, health, business promotion and creation of temporary employment. Besides the increase in expenditure, government revenue will also suffer due to the slow growth of the economy. The fiscal deficit in fiscal year 2003–04 will likely soar from $68 billion to close to $90 billion, or close to 7 percent of Hong Kong's GDP. Fortunately, Hong Kong has huge fiscal reserves of close to $300 billion. The one-time fiscal package of $11.8 billion has not done irreparable damage to Hong Kong's fiscal health, but it has interrupted the government's original budget plan to reduce the fiscal deficit.

The impact of SARS on trade is not yet apparent, as present exports are determined by orders in the pre-SARS period. Mainland's exports are still very competitive, with its exports going up by over 37 percent in May. However, SARS has adversely affected the ability of Hong Kong businesses to receive orders. For instance, the Swiss Jewelry and Watch Exhibition has prohibited the attendance of Hong Kong merchants. By May, SARS has affected 34 exhibitions scheduled in Hong Kong: 7 were cancelled and 27 were postponed to the fall or early next year (*Hong Kong Economic Journal*, 21 May 2003). With the lifting of the travel advisory to Hong Kong and Guangdong by the WHO in late May, it looks as if these exhibitions will go forward after postponement, and Hong Kong merchants should be able to make up for the bulk of lost orders in the fall. In late May, the government revised its 2003 export growth forecast from 6.6 percent to 5.5 percent. Growth of Mainland's trade has been very robust after Mainland's WTO entry, and the impact of SARS on Hong Kong's trade appears to be mild.

While the economic picture remains bleak in 2003, 2004 should herald full recovery. A weak US dollar should stimulate exports of the mainland and the region and would eventually pull Hong Kong out of the doldrums. ING Financial Markets forecast that Hong Kong's deflation would end in 2004, and property prices would also stabilize (*Hong Kong Commercial Daily*, 27 June 2003).

While the economic picture remains bleak in 2003, 2004 should herald full recovery.

Fallout on the Community

A narrow economic analysis cannot reflect the strong human face to the fallout from SARS. While the economic costs of SARS are more tangible, it is more difficult to estimate the social costs.

The initial reaction to the SARS outbreak in the Prince of Wales Hospital in mid-March was one of worry that the disease would spread to the community. The government's delay in acknowledging the risk of the spread and in taking strict quarantine measures to contain the spread has led to public confusion and a decline in confidence in the government. At the end of March, the large-scale outbreak of SARS cases in Amoy Gardens, a residential complex in urban Kowloon, caught the government unprepared for quarantine measures. Given the challenge of a deadly virus with unknown medium of environmental transmission, the confusing messages from the government and the experts could not inspire confidence in the public. Ignorance and paranoia have led to an exodus of residents from the infected residential blocks, and discriminatory protests by local residents against the setting up of quarantine camps in their districts. The government's indecision to suspend classes in all schools brought about fear and angry reactions from teachers and parents. Community surveys conducted during the months of March and April showed that around 31% to 40% of the respondents would not allow their children to go to school.[4] Without a clear voice from the government and the medical professionals, uncertainties increased people's anxiety and sense of helplessness.[5]

---

[4] "Second Survey on Hong Kong Public's Reactions and Attitudes to SARS", Press Release by Prof. Joseph Lau, Centre for Epidemiology and Biostatistics, The Chinese University of Hong Kong, May 27, 2003.
[5] "Survey Results on Public Responses to Atypical Pneumonia in Hong Kong", Press Release by Prof. Catherine Tang, Department of Psychology, The Chinese University of Hong Kong, March 20, 2003.

The jittery public fell prey to a teenage student's April Fools hoax on the Internet and rushed to supermarkets in panic shopping sprees to hoard food and household provisions on April 1. Homemakers carried the extra burden of childcare with students suspended from schools, increased household cleaning chores, and concern over their family members' health.[6] As the infection rate of frontline healthcare workers continued, frustrations of hospital staff climbed. Hospital staff complained about the inadequate provisions of protective measures and revealed the bureaucratic management of public hospitals. The fatality rate of healthcare workers and younger patients without chronic illness brought home the vulnerability of people to a dangerous disease. The realization that, despite its modern medical facilities, Hong Kong could not control SARS much better than the mainland is humbling. The pernicious conditions of public hygiene hidden behind the affluent facade of urban Hong Kong became exposed. The initial panic and anxiety turned to frustrations and anger. The majority of the public were dissatisfied with the way the government handled the SARS crisis.[3] In April, close to 60% of a random sample of respondents expressed dissatisfaction with the SAR government; dissatisfaction remained at 56% in May before the WHO travel advisory was lifted.[7]

Hong Kong's fall from grace was highlighted by the international community's rejection of its travelers. Once accustomed to its economic advantages, Hong Kong suffered the humiliation of being unwelcome. Some countries refused to grant visas to Hong Kong residents. Hong Kong merchants were barred from participating in international trade fairs. Students were turned away from overseas summer program. Even in mainland and Taiwan hotels, Hong Kong travelers were subjected to discriminatory practices. The collective victimization from unfair discrimination created a sense of helplessness.

With the majority of the population refraining from normal social activities, especially going out to crowded places,[4] the vibrant urban life was reduced to home confinement, either by choice or by quarantine. The imposed isolation of patients, their families, and healthcare workers rendered the battle against

---

[6] *"Survey on Stress from SARS for Hong Kong Women"*, YWCA Hong Kong, April 27, 2003.
[7] *"Public Opinion Poll on the SAR Government, May 2003: Highlights of the Results"*, Press Release by the Hong Kong Institute of Asia-Pacific Studies, The Chinese University of Hong Kong, May 26, 2003.

> ## The sudden and massive loss of human life brought grief not only to the family members, but also to close associates and vicariously to the public.

SARS a lonely course for those affected. The psychological impact of SARS is similar to other community disasters, which causes trauma and stress reactions. The sudden and massive loss of human life brought grief not only to the family members, but also to close associates and vicariously to the public who followed the daily news closely through the mass media. The death of healthcare workers was particularly traumatic. Surviving hospital staff suffered grief, guilt and anger from the loss. The public lamented the loss of society's talents. The distress of the survivors was less prominently portrayed in the media, though no less pervasive and damaging. Short-term and long-term stress reactions in the form of physical and psychological symptoms could be expected. Although many telephone hotlines have been initiated by social service agencies in response to the SARS crisis, the concerted effort to provide psychological intervention for the SARS crisis and its aftermath was not in place. The costs of care for the SARS induced and post-SARS stress reactions, as well as the costs to human resources arising from the stress reactions, need to be recognized. Some of the grief and anger reactions from the suffering and loss are turning into claims for compensation. The frustration of healthcare professionals is also reflected by their active participation in the protest march against the government on July 1, the sixth anniversary of Hong Kong's reunification with China.

The economic fallout exacerbates the collective gloom in the community. Financial loss due to SARS is experienced not only by patients' families, but also by people who lost their income due to the economic fallout. SARS struck a blow on the fledging recovery of the economy. Breadwinners were lost to the disease. Patients and their close contacts required to stay home for isolation worried about losing their jobs. Workers were asked to take no-pay leave. Businesses were closed due to the slump. These economic impacts on individuals and families form part of the SARS trauma.

Resilience of the Hong Kong Spirit

Out of crisis arise opportunities. The SARS fallout in Hong Kong has witnessed the resurgence of community values that have long been sidelined in favor of economic interests. Recognizing that they could depend on government intervention alone, individuals, groups, and organizations came up with their own initiatives to help, in cash and in kind. Four female senior officials of the government spearheaded a donation drive to set up funds for the future education of children orphaned by SARS. Other donations poured in for families of healthcare workers who lost their lives to SARS. Fund raising campaigns also targeted the improvement of protective measures for frontline healthcare workers and cleansing teams.

The civil society mobilized itself promptly. Many social service agencies and professional groups came forward to provide services for people affected by SARS. Hotlines were set up to provide counseling and support. Websites offered a range of information and resources, including guidelines for health protection and homework for school children via the Internet. Academics stepped outside of their ivory tower to address urgent medical, environmental, and social needs. The business sector promoted new products and strategies to stimulate local consumption. By the Easter holidays, the public has begun to return to active life. Local tours became a popular option for residents entrapped from their international travel restrictions. There is a common goal for the community. The sense of helplessness and isolation raised as concerns at the beginning of the crisis was later found to be less apparent among young people who noticed their interpersonal relationships have been strengthened during the process.[8]

A cross-sectoral group of community leaders initiated the Operation UNITE campaign to call upon everyone in the community to unite in strength to beat SARS by adopting a hygiene charter, organizing activities to lift community spirits and rebuild confidence, and to foster mutual care. Solidarity of the governmental and nongovernmental organizations as well as the business sectors was demonstrated. Open expressions of appreciation to the frontline

---

[8] *"Survey on the Impact of the SARS Incident on Interpersonal Relationship"*, YWCA Hong Kong, April 22, 2003.

A cross-sectoral group of community leaders initiated the Operation UNITE campaign to call upon everyone in the community to unite in strength to beat SARS by adopting a hygiene charter, organizing activities to lift community spirits and rebuild confidence, and to foster mutual care.

healthcare workers were spontaneous. Tributes were paid to the heroic professionalism of the frontline workers who valiantly sacrificed themselves to fight the disease.

The selfless service of medical staff who lost their lives in the battle against SARS was recognized. Their professionalism had earned widespread respect from the community. These role models provided Hong Kong with a revived sense of purpose and meaning, which had long been submerged under the pragmatic economic ethos of the Hong Kong, Inc. The jolt to the Hong Kong ego provided the HKSAR the opportunity to rebuild itself with a new identity and culture based on service, concern, and communality.

Opportunities for Hong Kong

Hong Kong aims to be an international service hub, and also a business center for the headquarters of multinational companies. This implies that Hong Kong has to strive for a very high quality sanitary environment and a superior healthcare system. An international service hub has to value human life above narrow business interests. Otherwise, the CEO's of multinationals would not find Hong Kong a hospitable base.

In the initial fight against SARS, the Hong Kong government has been slow to take quarantine measures, partly out of fear that such measures would have an adverse impact on the tourist industry. For example, despite the early warning of health professionals in Hong Kong, the government was reluctant to close the Prince of Wales Hospital after the alarming SARS outbreak there in early March, partly out of fear that it would alarm the public and the

> **The cooperation of Hong Kong and Guangdong medical experts has led to the discovery of the coronavirus as the cause of SARS. Hong Kong has also invited specialists in Chinese medicine to treat SARS patients.**

international community. During the SARS crisis, the Hong Kong government revealed an unsettling tendency to let narrow business interests set its priorities. This is partly because the constitution of the HKSAR is structured in such a way that business interests dominate its polity. Unfortunately for Hong Kong, these narrow business interests had downplayed the essentials of public health.

For post-SARS reparation, the Hong Kong government has set up two task forces, one led by the Financial Secretary to revive the Hong Kong economy, and the other led by the Chief Secretary to clean up Hong Kong. To ensure sustainability and effectiveness of these efforts, the government should take on board lessons learned from the SARS crisis. SARS has highlighted Hong Kong's symbiosis with China, and its interconnectedness with the international community. In the new era of globalization, strategic planning should adopt a global and multidimensional frame of mind. Health and economics are not just local issues. Their solutions cannot be limited to the responsibility of the government. The resilient Hong Kong spirit and the vast pool of human resources are gold mines that could be tapped to cultivate a revived HKSAR.

SARS has also led some proponents to advocate a slow down in Hong Kong's economic integration with Guangdong. Some even suggested sealing the border with the mainland to fight SARS. However, the Taiwanese experience with strict quarantine of mainland and Hong Kong travelers has been shown to be a failure. Taiwan-Mainland links are too close for strict quarantine to work. As Hong Kong-Mainland links are much closer than Taiwan-Mainland links, sealing off of the Hong Kong-Mainland border cannot possibly work. Sealing the border is objectionable not only on economic grounds, but also on the grounds of human rights: Hong Kong residents have over half a million children or spouse living in the mainland.

Instead of slowing down Hong Kong-Guangdong integration, deep integration with Guangdong will be a more effective strategy to fight SARS. Hitherto, the mainland was only interested in economic integration with the world. Non-economic areas were off limits. However, the disastrous cover-up of SARS exacerbated the outbreak of the disease in China, and the Chinese leadership changed its attitude. Beijing now accepts WHO rules on public health and disease control, and China is planning to build a modern Center for Disease Control (CDC) in anticipation of the 2008 Olympics. Hong Kong should press for cooperation with the mainland not only on economic issues, but also on public health, disease control, sanitation, environmental and social issues. The benefits of close collaboration are encouraging. For example, the cooperation of Hong Kong and Guangdong medical experts has led to the discovery of the coronavirus as the cause of SARS. Hong Kong has also invited specialists in Chinese medicine to treat SARS patients in Hong Kong, and the treatment has shown encouraging results.

On 30 June 2003, Hong Kong and the mainland signed a free-trade agreement, officially known as the CEPA (Closer Economic Partnership Arrangement). Hong Kong products would enjoy tariff-free access to the mainland market, and more importantly, many service industries would enjoy favorable access to the mainland market. While the CEPA was conceived in the pre-SARS era, Beijing has reportedly sweetened the deal for Hong Kong to help the SARS-ravaged Hong Kong economy (*Ming Pao*, 17 June 2003). The deal is a landmark in the economic integration of Hong Kong and the mainland. In the field of public health, the deal allows joint-ventures in hospitals and clinics, and also allows doctors outside the mainland to provide short term medical services in the mainland after approval by mainland's health authority. The CEPA is likely to strengthen the budding cooperation in medicine and health between mainland and Hong Kong

In the near future, south China will continue to be a hotbed for new viruses. Hong Kong will be a strategic base for the monitoring and control of such viruses due to its location and capability in modern medical research. As a window of China, Hong Kong is unique not only in terms of its geography and connectivity, but also in terms of its modernity, transparency, and free media. Hong Kong journalists were the first to report on the outbreak of SARS in Guangdong despite the initial cover-up of the authorities. Hong Kong could be a catalyst for development in the mainland, not only in economic matters,

> # If we learn from our lessons, the 2003 SARS crisis could be remembered as a watershed for the new identity of the HKSAR.

but also in issues of public health, sanitation, and the environment. These processes of reintegration with the mainland provide new directions for Hong Kong's positioning in the One-Country-Two Systems framework.

On the local front, post-SARS rebuild policies should look beyond putting in place an infrastructure and a model of preparedness for future crises. Sustaining community care and concern with the current moral high ground will enhance the effectiveness of future campaigns to foster civic mindedness and to improve public health and personal hygiene in Hong Kong. Witnessing the human costs of SARS in an interconnected world impresses an emotional memory that propels learning and action. The SARS epidemic demonstrates how individuals' personal hygiene and habits are linked to environmental and health risks. It illustrates how the local and global communities are closely connected. The community witnessed first-hand the experiences of suffering, loss, and discrimination. It also revisited the meaning of service, sacrifice, and sharing.

Rebuilding Hong Kong's economy and hygiene requires not only an infrastructure of systems and laws. To make it sustainable, it should be grounded in an ethos of human values that recognize interdependence and give purpose to living. It should also recognize the psychosocial responses that create crises and opportunities. The vast resource of energy from the community, the service orientation of professionals and frontline workers, and the expertise of local academics could be tapped in more strategic and coordinated efforts. These opportunities should not be missed.

It is probable that the HKSAR will catch SARS or another new epidemic again. However, if we learn from our lessons, the 2003 SARS crisis could be remembered as a watershed for the new identity of the HKSAR.

YUN-WING SUNG

Dr. Yun-Wing Sung is currently Chairman and Professor of the Economics Department, and Associate Director of the Hong Kong Institute of Asia-Pacific Studies at The Chinese University of Hong Kong. He is also Editor of the *Asian Economic Journal*, Book Review Editor of *Pacific Economic Review*, and Corresponding Editor of *Asian Pacific Economic Literature*. He obtained his Ph.D. in Economics from the University of Minnesota in 1979. He was Research Fellow at the Australian National University in 1985, Visiting Scholar at the University of Chicago in 1985, at Harvard-Yenching Institute at Harvard University in 1989–90, and at University of Nottingham in 1996. His research interests cover international trade and economic development in China, Hong Kong, and Taiwan. He has authored eight books, edited four books, and published numerous articles in the area.

Major Publications:

Books:

The China-Hong Kong Connection: The Key to China's Open Door Policy, Cambridge University Press, Cambridge, 1991, 183 pages.
The Fifth Dragon: The Emergence of the Pearl River Delta (coauthored wtih P.W. Liu, Richard Wong, and P.K. Lau), Addison-Wesley, Singapore, 1995, 259 pages.
Hong Kong and South China: The Economic Synergy, City University Press, Hong Kong, 1988, 181 pages.

Articles:

"The role of Hong Kong in China's export drive", *Australian Journal of Chinese Affairs*, No. 15, pp. 83–101, 1986.
"China's economic reform I: The debates in China", *Asian-Pacific Economic Literature*, Vol. I, No. 1, pp. 1–25, 5.1987 (lead article of issue), (co-authored with Thomas M.H. Chan).

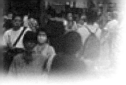

"China's impact on the Asian Pacific regional economy", in *Bus. Contemp. World*, 5(2): 105–128, 1993.

"The Hong Kong economy through the 1997 barrier", *Asian Survey* **37**(8): 705–719, 1997.

"Growth of Hong Kong before and after its reversion to China: The China factor", *Pacific Economic Review* **5**(2): 201–228, 2000 (co-authored with Wong Kar-yiu).

"Costs and benefits of export-oriented foreign investment: The case of China", *Asian Economic Journal* **14**(1): 55–70, 2001.

"Gender wage differentials and occupational segregation in Hong Kong, 1981–1996", *Pacific Economic Review* **6**(3): 345–359, 2001 (coauthored with Junsen Zhang and Chi-Shing Chan).

FANNY M. CHEUNG

Dr. Fanny Cheung is Professor of Psychology and Chairperson of the Department of Psychology, The Chinese University of Hong Kong, where she has taught since 1977. From 1996–1999, she took leave from the University to serve as the founding Chairperson of the Equal Opportunities Commission of Hong Kong. At the Chinese University, she has been Dean of the Faculty of Social Science. She pioneered the field of gender studies in Hong Kong by founding the Gender Research Programme in 1985. She also initiated the Gender Studies Programmes at the graduate and undergraduate level in mid 1990s. She is currently Director of the Gender Research Centre at the Chinese University. She has also established the Assessment and Training Centre as a joint effort between the Department of Psychology and the Faculty of Business Administration to promote evidence-based practice in assessment to organizations.

Dr. Cheung was a past President of the Hong Kong Psychological Society (1984–85) and a past President of the Division of Clinical and Community Psychology of the International Association of Applied Psychology (1990–94). Her research interests include personality assessment, and psychopathology among the Chinese people, violence against women, and gender equality. She has developed the Chinese (Cross-Cultural) Personality Assessment Inventory, an indigenous personality measure appropriate for the Asian cultural context. Her academic publications include 7 books and over 100 journal articles, chapters and monographs. She is currently co-editing a Special Section on Psychological Assessment in Asian Countries for the international journal, *Psychological Assessment*.

Dr. Cheung has served in many government committees and advisory bodies. For her contributions to the community, she was awarded the Badge of Honor in 1986, appointed as Justice of Peace in 1988 and awarded the Honor of Officer of the Most Excellent Order of the British Empire (OBE) in 1997.

Contact details:
Fanny M. Cheung, Ph.D.
Professor of Psychology and Chairperson
Department of Psychology
The Chinese University of Hong Kong
E-mail: fmcheung@cuhk.edu.hk

9

Will SARS Result in a Financial Crisis? — Differentiating Real, Transient, and Permanent Economic Effects of a Health Crisis

by *FRANK T. LORNE*

All financial crises are preceded by some deteriorating economic conditions. However, deteriorating conditions alone will not cause a crisis. It is a set of deteriorating conditions being sped up by some additional conditions that could develop into a financial crisis. These conditions include: (a) a lack of liquidity, (b) an increase in moral hazard problems, and (c) an increase in adverse selection problems. This essay formulates a theoretical foundation upon which economic policies for SARS should be built.

A deteriorating economic condition by itself does not constitute a crisis, although it could certainly constitute a reduction in wealth. Technically speaking, economists would say that an economy's production possibility frontier could be shifting inward, due to natural disasters and what not. But as long as the economy stays on the production possibility frontier, perhaps doing more of some things and less of other things, economic efficiency will not be affected. Bad luck caused a one-shot price adjustment, but will not cause a continuous deteriorating spill-over effect into real sector and the financial sector of an economy. The main proposition this essay wishes to pursue is the following: economic policies dealing with SARS should focus on these three conditions, recognizing a difference between transient effects and permanent effects while also noticing that transient effects could, through mismanagement of the three conditions, lead to permanent effects. If the three conditions cannot be managed appropriately, the result will not only cause an economy to move from one point of the production possibility frontier to another, but could very well cause an the economy to be INSIDE its production frontier, with the effects of an emerging financial crisis feeding back into the real operations of an economy. Such is the real cost of a crisis.

2003 may be an unfortunate year for China in that a health epidemic caused by a virus called Severe Acute Respiratory Syndrome (SARS) hit the region. The event, at its face value, has no bearings on financial crisis as it is primarily a health crisis. Yet, because the nature of the disease was not well known, particularly at the initial stage of the crisis, panic and worry could possibly lead to an economic deterioration. The effects of SARS on the economy is intellectually interesting in that the epidemic affects two of the three conditions above directly, and thus open up the possibilities that a health crisis could conceivably lead to a financial crisis. The immediate effects of SARS on the real economy during the early stages of the crisis had been obvious: the hardest hit sectors being airline, tourism, and retailing. Empty shopping malls, transportation hubs, restaurants and hotels have all been the vivid images of the immediate effects of SARS.

The real effects of SARS, however, should be analyzed both from a short-run and a long run effect, with the long run effects being contingent upon how the short-run effects are being remedied. Sectoral shifts from retail, food, traveling towards supermarkets, household products, toiletries and pharmaceutical products are generally observed, but it is not yet clear whether the shift is transient or permanent. A report on SCMP, May 7, 2003, suggested that as far as Hong Kong is concerned, the effects need not be perceived as permanent, and even if permanent, it may not be vulnerable: Visitor spending as a percentage of GDP in Hong Kong is not large. Estimated to be 6.1%, it is slightly more than Singapore's 5%, but less than Malaysia's 7.1%. The percentages in mainland China and Taiwan could be even smaller. Vulnerability in terms of consumption, measured by consumption as a percentage of GDP, also is not high (56% in Hong Kong, compared with a high figures of 70% in Indonesia and the Philippines). If one counts the whole travel, tourism and restaurant business of Hong Kong as a percentage of GDP (HK$1.32 trillion), it amounts to about 9% (HK$120 billion). From this, the SCMP article estimated that a short-run effect on the Hong Kong economy will be around HK$40 billion. On this score, the government's rescue relief of HK$11.8 billion seemed comparable and sensible.

Yet, there are reasons to believe that the Hong Kong government's consideration is inadequate, or not comprehensive enough. At the outside, we have to admit that until the short-run effects are back to normal, or if unlucky, unavoidably settling to a new equilibrium and thus becoming permanent, whether a health crisis could trigger a financial crisis remains to be the question. Indeed, to the extent that financial crisis can also impact on permanent shifts in the economy, the need for discussing the possible origin of a crisis, and how to prevent it, may all come to play beyond what a short-run economic relief package could accomplish.

The critical problem caused by SARS is an increase in risk and uncertainty of people's daily activities, affecting the way people interact with each other, increasing what economists would label as a class of asymmetric information problems. To be sure, if SARS did not exist, society has already been organized in certain ways that had provided assurance on the normal risk people usually face. For examples, brand names, business practices, people's living habits, have been structured in a way to alleviate a "normal" risk perception level of human and business interactions. But whatever that level of assurance a society or a community has been carrying, it may not be high enough to cope with the extra asymmetric information caused by SARS, or at least not until the

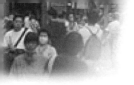

roots of the asymmetric information is somehow reduced or controlled. Using the terminology of this essay, for moral hazard, people will be worrying about who had used what, when and where, and whether the person you will be shaking hands with are carrying germs around him/her. For adverse selection, people will shy away from new contacts and concentrate on dealing with people and things they are familiar of dealing with in the past. If the medical war on SARS is not fought effectively, these asymmetric information problem will continue to affect all aspects of community and business activities, turning a health crisis into not only effects on the economy sectorally, but generally, affecting financial transactions as well.

The way a higher risk and uncertainty can affect financial transactions is more subtle, but with a ripple and repercussion effects much larger than that of a sectoral impact. Understandably, stocks of airlines, fast food chain stores, tourism, retail clothing stores had been hard hit. These stock prices may be passively affected by earning perception, but can actively affect investors' perception as well. Already, the general risk perceptions of all companies seem to be affected. Aside from delaying projects, temporarily shutting down not only business but manufacturing facilities (e.g. Beijing staff of Motorola sent home), there were reports of delayed payment of dividends of company policies, hiring schemes put on hold, capital expenditure plans and advertising campaigns halted, and new funds scheduled to be launched put on hold. Asian large supply chain import-exporter, Li & Fung, reporting international customers canceling shopping trips to the area, also revealed that there are some source switching from China to elsewhere (from various reports on SCMP, May 7–3, 2003).

It is difficult to tell how earnings of companies have been significantly affected yet, as they are unlikely to be detected until a few months later. Although the Hong Kong stock market price-earning ratio amid the health crisis is still considered to low (11.9 compared to 16.4 in Taiwan, and 40 in some western countries of the world), and alleged by fund managers soliciting buying interests, Hong Kong market is essentially trading at 0.87 times its book value. Yet, there is no assurance that book value of a company will not be further revised downward. Certainly, a temporary recovery of the stock market on a daily basis cannot be interpreted as any indication of a market rationalization of the real situations. Indeed, it could be the result of market participants trading base on asymmetric information. On the day Shanghai and Shenzhen stock exchanges re-opened after an extended shut-down, an initial rally could be quickly eroded by traders talks such as "lingering worries over when the Sars outbreak will be brought under control".

Financial markets are particularly vulnerable to asymmetric information. These possibilities are likely to be prominent as earning reports are gradually disclosed. SCMP, May 10, 2003 reported that company directors are so far cautious about buy-back opportunities, when previous come-back for September 11 was compared. Directors generally believed the diseases will have "profound impact" on earnings. Two effects are possible: (a) the market is likely to become more volatile, as traders will capitalize on every bit of information, rumors or not. (b) If trading values are consistently below book values, it would suggest that the book values should be revised downward. Both effects suggested that the market value of firms doing business in the area, if SARS is not effectively controlled within a reasonable short period, could be further lowered because of asymmetric information. The effects of these downward revisions not only can affect the stock values of companies, but could have spill over effects on banking portfolios as well.

In principle, a financial crisis of a short term nature can be quickly eliminated by appropriately handling the first factor of the three conditions mentioned, i.e. an increase in liquidity. In Hong Kong, indeed, we saw the market bouncing back in May, preceded perhaps by a series of companies' buy-back program of their own stocks. The same applies to banks requiring a larger loan loss reserve in case bad debt continues. Yet, an implementation of a liquidity rescue policy could be itself subject to problems of asymmetric information. That is, those who are in need of loans are those that are in the worst shape. Certainly, a continuation of SARS spread will provide a good excuse for spreading moral hazards of various kinds in terms of an exaggeration of transient conditions and various misuses of short-run relief as well. If these problems are not anticipated and appropriately curbed, financial crisis could erupt.

The analysis above suggests the possibility of having an over zealous remedy of liquidity that could itself leads to the possibility of a crisis. If the source of the problem is an increase in risk and uncertainty, an increase in problems related to asymmetric information, the cure for the problem may indeed has to be focused on these dimensions. The key to controlling a health-induced financial crisis is on how asymmetric information problems caused by the

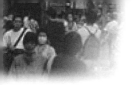

health crisis can be reduced. In this respect, it cannot be argued that asymmetric information problems related to SARS have been handled most effectively; not can it be considered purely as a local issue. Indeed, because Hong Kong's economy depends heavily on import and export trade, Pearl River Delta in particular, and the greater China region in general, how successful the health crisis can be curbed, and how successful the financial spill-overs can be prevented could depend on how the region as a whole is handling the situation. Pearl River Delta is of strategic importance for both Hong Kong and the Greater China, because this area was rumored to be the origin of SARS. Insofar that reducing risk and uncertainty requires ascertaining the root of the problem, scientific verification of the cause of the disease, people's diet, living habits, etc. all could contribute to people's understanding of the health crisis, and thus help to alleviate the risk and uncertainty in daily decision problems of where to go, whom to interact, etc. These problems could be compounded at a junction when Hong Kong is closed to being lifted off WHO's travel warning list, information concerning how Guangdong has been handling the crisis is still scattered, with rumors that reporters and WHO's staff have been barred from on-site communications with the outside world (see "Media being kept in the dark in Guangdong, SCMP, May 12, 2003, A3). Although problems in Beijing are allegedly under control, Taiwan is experiencing its highest daily infection rate as the day of this writing.

If there is anything that can be learned from the 1998 Asian financial crisis, it is that it was, like an epidemic, contagious. Thus, even if Hong Kong is found to have zero infection rate, if problems elsewhere is not controlled and indeed in the worst scenario, developed into a financial crisis, Hong Kong economic condition cannot be spared. The long run effects of SARS remain to be explored. This essay points out some underlying essential parameters for further considerations. A *bandage* solution, whether administered locally in Hong Kong, or regionally in Pearl River Delta, or even the Greater China, could only exasperate rather than alleviate the problem.

FRANK T. LORNE

Dr. Lorne graduated from the University of Washington with a Ph.D. degree in economics in 1978. He has over 20 years of university research and teaching experience in North America and Asia. A summary of his professional experience is given below:

Professional and Education Consulting

·   Development of Continued Education Courses on Business and Economics, 2000 to present.
·   Assisted organizing conferences on East-West Trade issues, technology transfers, and venture capital, 1988 to present.
·   Participated in projects on "Technology Markets", University of Science and Technology, China, 1986; organized Asian Venture Capital Institute Seminar, 1997 (first time in PRC); development of courses on "Business Culture in China", 1999 to present.

Other Professional Work

·   Production of MBA Educational Video and Internet development, 1999- present.
·   Research on Sustainable Development (with Lawrence Lai), The University of Hong Kong, 1999-present.
·   Analysis of Insurance Industry, with Center of Economic Research, Hong Kong, 1995–1997.
·   Asian Business Association, Los Angeles (Board of Directors, 1994). Networked with Business Leaders. Helped formulate a position paper for the Association.
·   Victor Valley Economic Development Association, Marketing Committee.
    Evaluated economic impact and suggested alternatives for regional development, 1991–1993.

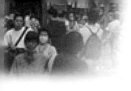

- International Regional Development, deal source, marketing, design and coordination of projects.

Entrepreneurial Activities

- Large format (IMAX) project development, 1994–1997.
- Educational Tour, 1998–2000.

Contact Address: **#1803-1239 West Georgia Street,**
Vancouver, B.C., V6E 4R8
Tel: (604) 899-4518
E-mail: askmefrank@yahoo.com

10

Facing the Unknowns of SARS in Hong Kong

by *Kwok-yung Yuen* and *Malik Peiris*

For good or ill, the media today has weaved itself into the fabric of all public affairs. Thus it was hardly surprising that in February 2003, people in Hong Kong learned about an outbreak of atypical pneumonia in the nearby Guangdong province from newspapers rather than from official channels. Later, as the initial rumors and confusion cleared away, the World Health Organization labeled the novel, or new, atypical pneumonia syndrome, Severe Acute Respiratory Syndrome, or SARS. Within a week of the first newspaper reports, the Hong Kong government convened a panel of experts to study the contingency of a Guangdong-like outbreak in Hong Kong, and to begin the surveillance of severe pneumonia. At that time, hospital surveillance in the territory did not reveal any increase in the number of severe community acquired pneumonia.

Unfortunately, due to the "one country two systems" mode of governance, official channels of communication between Hong Kong and Guangdong were

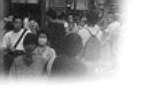

not well established. Indeed, during those early stages, the media were the main source of information about developments in the mainland.

The limited information we could piece together from newspapers and official bulletins was quite alarming. For example, an astonishing 105 out of the initial 305 cases of the novel atypical pneumonia involved relatively young and healthy hospital workers. This pointed to an unusually virulent intra-hospital spread of the disease. Infections within families were also alarmingly common.

Each year, during winter and early spring, influenza and secondary bacterial infection of the lungs are the most common causes of hospital admissions for respiratory tract illness. It became quickly evident that the standard arsenal of antibacterial and antiviral agents used to fight influenza was not working well at all against this new disease. We had no official surveillance records on atypical pneumonia from the mainland, but the mortality figure of 5 in 305 could not be considered as low if the patients were mainly young, healthy adults. The outbreak in Guangdong was ominous. We started to ponder and strategize on ways to solve this mystery.

The differentiation of typical and atypical pneumonia is difficult, if data on clinical syndromes, microbiological analyses, and patients' response to the penicillin group of antibiotics are not available. These we did not have at that time. In general, typical pneumonia has a very acute onset of fever, chills, chest pains, increased respiratory rate, and cough with rusty sputum caused by pus forming bacteria. Blood counts usually show an increase in the type of white blood cells called neutrophils. Patients of typical pneumonia respond very well to the penicillin group of antibiotics. So pathogens behind typical pneumonia such as *Streptococcus pneumoniae*, *Haemophilus influenzae* and *Staphylococcus aureus* are unlikely to be the cause of major outbreaks in hospital settings where antibiotics are liberally prescribed.

Atypical pneumonia usually presents less acute upper respiratory tract symptoms. The cough is usually dry. Blood counts may show either increased or normal white blood cells. Accordingly, findings from clinical examination are often disproportionate to more severe changes revealed by chest X-rays.

Atypical pneumonia is mainly caused by five different bacterial agents and other less common respiratory viruses. One clear signal of atypical pneumonia is that patients do not respond to treatment with the penicillin group of antibiotics. This group of antibiotics destroys bacteria by inhibiting

Rumors multiplied as the media reported more deaths of relatively young patients, including doctors and nurses. Panic buying of vinegar and certain traditional Chinese herbal cures ensued.

the rebuilding of bacterial cell walls; and Mycoplasma pneumoniae, the most common cause of atypical pneumonia do not have cell walls. Moreover, penicillin does not penetrate infected cells very well and other atypical pneumonia is predominantly caused by intracellular pathogens such as Chlamydia pneumoniae, Chlamydiae psittasci, Coxiella burnetti and Legionella pneumophila which often hide inside the human cell.

Though the Guangdong outbreak appeared to be atypical pneumonia, the actual culprit was not known. This was a major community acquired outbreak with a significant mortality even in young patients, and a high frequency of transmission to hospital staff. As far as we could tell, the five bacterial agents normally associated with atypical pneumonia were unlikely candidates. Moreover, all these bacterial agents are often associated with a specific antibody response in patients and could be easily diagnosed by any standard microbiology laboratory. So we concluded quite early that the cause was viral.

Rumors multiplied as the media reported more deaths of relatively young patients, including doctors and nurses. Panic buying of vinegar and certain traditional Chinese herbal cures ensued. People believed that vapor from boiling vinegar cleansed the air of bacteria, while the herbs detoxified the body and dissipated "heat" in the system caused by infection.

Looking back, such behavior may not be as bizarre as they appeared. Young medical workers dying one after another in hospital settings belonged in the dim past before antibiotics came on the scene and changed all the rules of treating infectious diseases. Such scenarios had not been seen for 30 years. Panic was almost inevitable.

Hong Kong was relatively tranquil compared with the commotion gripping Guangdong. This seems quite typical of explosive epidemics: there is always a lull before the storm. Then the invasion started. The index, or first, patient of the Hong Kong outbreak, and probably the global epidemic, was one Dr. Liu JL,

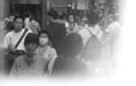

a professor of nephrology from a teaching hospital in Guangzhou. He had had contact with patients suffering from atypical pneumonia and then developed a fever and cough, which was treated by antibiotics (penicillin and ofloxacin) five days before visiting Hong Kong. Within 24 hours of checking in, he had infected more than 10 people staying in the same hotel.

Dr. Liu was admitted to Kwong Wah Hospital in Kowloon, Hong Kong, where he deteriorated rapidly. Warded in the intensive care unit, he was intubated and ventilated (breathing assisted by respirator). He had fever and the chest X-ray showed a diffuse fine mottling (a type of opacity) which suggested viral pneumonia. His blood count was low and he had to be ventilated with a high concentration of oxygen to sustain life. Antibiotics, which should cure both bacterial pneumonia and atypical bacterial pneumonia, were administered, but were not working. KYY was invited by Dr. Andrew Yip and Dr. Chi-leung Watt, both medical officers at Kwong Wah, to participate in the treatment. KYY initiated a course of Ribavirin, a broad-spectrum antiviral agent, which is effective against respiratory, hepatitic, and hemorrhagic fever viruses. Additionally, the patient was given steroid as a final effort to reduce the form of lung damage called ARDS (acute respiratory distress syndrome).

He continued to deteriorate and died two weeks after admission. No bacteria, virus, fungus or parasite could be found in his respiratory secretions, blood, or other body fluids. Basically we failed to save him and also failed to make a microbiological diagnosis.

Soon after the index patient died, his brother-in-law, Mr. Chan YP, was admitted to Kwong Wah Hospital for exactly the same condition. We see this as a turning point. That a member of the family was infected by the same mysterious illness settled any doubts that we had a real crisis on our hands.

In view of our failure with the previous patient, it seemed that the only way to deal with the mystery was to extract lung tissue from this new patient before he received any anti-microbial treatment. This was an extremely invasive surgical procedure to perform on a sick patient. After thorough consideration led by Dr. Andrew Wong, Chief of Service in Medicine, the operation was performed and the lung tissue sent to the Queen Mary Hospital, the teaching hospital of The University of Hong Kong, for microbiological analysis.

Now we set out to unravel the mystery. Most discoveries are made through educated guesses plus trial and error. We started by going through the list of

> **An antigenic shift describes a dramatic antigenic change associated with the reshuffling of virus genes called gene reassortment leading to a virus that cannot be contained by existing strategies. Such a shift is witnessed once in 20 to 50 years and is associated with very high morbidity and mortality.**

all the DNA and RNA[1] viruses that are associated with respiratory illnesses (doctors call this the list of differential diagnoses). We virtually started "blind," but this was the winding and many-branched road that finally led us to the culprit.

As we were in late winter and early spring, influenza was very high on every one's mental line-up as a possible solution. Moreover, one died and two others in the same family of five had recently returned from Fujian province (also in south China) with the avian influenza A H5N1. Thus, for a time, our attention was skewed towards the possibility of an emerging avian influenza virus with the ability to spread from human to human, and which may herald a global epidemic.

The other possibility high on our list of differential diagnoses was an antigenically drifted human influenza, which typically happens every few years. An antigenic drift describes a slight mutation that is not difficult to control. Antigenic drift is the reason why (to be properly protected against influenza) the elderly should receive a different prophylactic flu vaccine injection each year.

Subsequently, we considered the much more frightening possibility of an antigenically shifted human influenza A (the most virulent type of influenza). An antigenic shift describes a dramatic antigenic change associated with the reshuffling of virus genes called gene reassortment leading to a virus that

---

[1] DNA and RNA are cellular materials that carry genetic information and instructions for replication. Human cells use DNA. Viruses may use either DNA or RNA.

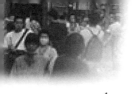

cannot be contained by existing strategies. Such a shift is witnessed once in 20 to 50 years and is associated with very high morbidity and mortality.

Though influenza was high on our list of differential diagnoses, a number of factors argued firmly against pursuing this line of thought. Our viral cultures optimized for influenza, genetic tests, and antigen tests had so far uniformly returned negative for influenza. Moreover, our patients did not respond to antiviral drugs tailor made for influenza, such as the amantadine and oseltamivir. In this light, other viruses than influenza with the potential of causing an outbreak had to be carefully considered. We had six possible candidates in mind: the *adenovirus, parainfluenza viruses, respiratory syncytial virus, metapneumovirus, rhinovirus*, and *coronaviruses*. Of these, only the *adenovirus* (besides the *influenza virus*) is a common cause of severe pneumonia among young, healthy adults. It seemed very unlikely that the others could be associated with the kind of acute symptoms that we were witnessing.

Moreover, further genetic testing of infected tissues by reverse transcription — polymerase chain reaction (RT-PCR) and PCR[2] or antigen testing, turned out negative for most of these viruses except for the *adenovirus*. So the *adenovirus* came into sharp focus. However, our initial enthusiasm was soon dismissed by a subsequent finding: when we compared the proportion of adenovirus DNA in the nasopharyngeal secretions of SARS patients with that in normal individuals, we found no difference. Evidently, the DNA of this virus could be detected in many normal individuals (perhaps from previous infections). So we were back to square one: if influenza was not the culprit, then what was?

We do not have at hand a good genetic or antigen test for coronavirus at this stage in time. But after excluding influenza and adenovirus, the conventional viruses that may cause a clinical picture such as this, we now have to consider a possible novel viral antigen. We try out a number of molecular tests to pick up novel viruses, including low stringency PCR and RT-PCR and random primer RT-PCR.

---

[2] RT-PCR and PCR are standard laboratory techniques that greatly multiply sections of genetic material (up to billions of copies from just a single copy) from diseased tissues in order to tease out pathogens. RT-PCR is used for RNA viruses such as the coronavirus, while PCR is used for DNA viruses such as the adenovirus.

Our colleague, Dr. Chan Kwok Hung was encouraged to try as many new cell lines (animal cells as medium for viral culture) as possible, beyond the standard four or five that were normally used.

What we needed next were luck and lots of patience.

One of the cell lines Chan chose comprised embryonic monkey kidney cells, a cell previously shown in our own lab to have the ability to sustain the growth of a range of respiratory viruses. The use of this cell line (FRhk-4) was probably the most important decision in the discovery of the pathogen behind SARS. The lung tissue of Mr. Chan YP (the brother-in-law of the index patient) was inoculated into this cell line for viral culture together with other specimens from patients with pneumonia associated with recent travel to Guangdong. Miraculously, significant changes were observed in this cell line. In a healthy cell line, rectangular cells are packed tile-like, looking almost like a brick wall. When infection occurs, cells separate from the tiled pattern and take on circular shapes. We saw detachment and rounding up through the microscope! This is called a cytopathic effect, which suggests the destruction of the cell line due to the presence of a virus. This occurred with the lung biopsy specimen of Mr Chan YP as well as another patient with SARS-like pneumonia. However, such cytopathic effects can also be caused by toxic substances in the specimen or by adventitious agents such as mycoplasms. To rule out mycoplasma, a very common contaminant of laboratory cultures, DNA sequencing by multiple PCR using eight sets of consensus primers was carried out. These returned negative, so mycoplasma was definitely ruled out.

The infected cell line was then used to test for antibodies both from infected patients and normal individuals. Since blood serum from healthy individuals would not contain the relevant antibody, nothing would happen whether they are applied to normal or infected cell lines. However, blood serum from a SARS patient (with the relevant antibody) would show reaction when applied to an infected cell line, if the culture in our laboratory was indeed the pathogen behind SARS. This reaction is detected by staining the antibodies with a fluorescent compound. Within a few days, we successfully set up the fluorescent antibody assay for testing of patients' serum.

While all this was happening, Dr. John Nicholls from the Department of Pathology had successfully observed the viral particles both in the infected cell line and the patient's lung tissue. We were now sure that there was indeed

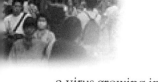

a virus growing in the cells. Help was also secured from Dr. Wilima Lim, head of the government virus unit who kindly supplied us with paired sera[3] for the confirmation of antibody response. She also helped us to do negative stained[4] electron microscopy for the confirmation of the size and morphology (shape) of SARS *coronavirus*.

We had now shown that a coronavirus could be isolated from a SARS patient and the patient had mounted a specific antibody response that reacted to the infected cell line in our laboratory. Serum from normal blood donors and patients suffering from other types of pneumonia did not have antibody response against this infected cell line.

But the next important question was whether this coronavirus was a novel one or just one of the 13 known coronaviruses found in human or animals. Dr. Leo Poon did a random PCR on the infected and un-infected cell lines (this means that sections of DNA from cell lines were multiplied, or amplified, numerous times and compared) using the same primers and conditions. Any unique fragments of gene amplified from an infected cell line which is absent in an un-infected cell line were fished out. This gene fishing exercise was rewarding. We identified a unique fragment of gene of 646 base pairs, which encoded part of the RNA replicase gene of this SARS coronavirus. By matching this DNA sequence with other known coronaviruses, we could determine whether this was a known or novel coronavirus. The closest match from this fragment of gene was to viruses within the family coronavirus confirming our electron microscopic observations. However, the sequence only had distant similarity to known coronaviruses. Leo therefore concluded that we were probably dealing with a novel coronavirus.

We had now set about developing two important tools in diagnosing SARS (a first big step in the fight against any new infectious disease): the antibody test, and a RT-PCR test designed by using the genetic information from the 646 base pairs. Using the clinical specimens from SARS patients from the three different hospitals in Hong Kong, we were able to demonstrate that 45 out of 50 SARS patients returned positive in either or both of these diagnostic

---

[3] "Pair sera" refers to blood serum collected from a patient on the day of admission and 18 days after admission.

[4] "Negative stained" refers to a procedure in which the surrounding material rather than the viral material is stained for the purpose of observation.

Our preliminary diagnostic tools had proven effective.

tests. These 50 patients had fever of 38 degree Celsius or more, cough or shortness of breath, and a new shadow on chest X-rays. They did not respond to antibiotic treatment for typical and atypical pneumonia nor had a history of epidemiological exposure to SARS (they had been in contact with other SARS infected persons or environment). In summary, all 50 patients who tested positive also fulfilled the WHO criteria for the diagnosis of SARS.

Our preliminary diagnostic tools had proven effective.

KYY, being a member of the government's expert panel for the outbreak, all our findings were communicated within hours to senior medical and health officials so that they could formulate preventive and treatment strategies.

Through regular teleconferencing between Malik Peiris and the WHO network of laboratories coordinated by Klaus Stohr of WHO, information was disseminated to all interested parties within the shortest possible time.

Our first isolate from the open lung biopsy was available almost immediately to researchers worldwide. We announced this discovery on 22 March 2003 at a press conference. The credibility of our discovery was later confirmed when it was published in *Lancet*, a highly respected medical journal.

During the outbreak in Hong Kong, we had the valuable opportunity of tending to SARS patients in seven acute hospitals. We are deeply thankful to all the consultants and other healthcare workers from the departments of medicine, intensive care, and clinical microbiology in these hospitals who patiently discussed cases with us and also interacted with us on the management of those patients. They even allowed us to use clinical and laboratory data for analysis and publication in *Lancet*. So after numerous hours of prospective clinical data and specimen collection, laboratory test running and statistical analysis, we managed to submit our first two papers to *Lancet* within one month of the announcement of our discovery.

We must make it clear that teamwork was fundamental to our success. Every author of these two *Lancet* papers contributed significantly to different aspects of the work: from clinical bedside management, through laboratory microbiology and virology, to molecular biology and histopathology. The first paper was about Coronavirus as a possible cause of severe acute respiratory

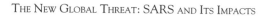
> # Finding the responsible virus and defining the syndrome of SARS are just the beginning of a long and difficult journey, which we hope will culminate in the effective treatment and prevention of SARS.

syndrome (*Lancet*: 2003 Apr 19; **361**(9366):1319–1325). The second was on the clinical progression and viral load (the density of viral presence) in a community outbreak of coronavirus-associated SARS pneumonia: a prospective study (*Lancet*. 2003 May 24; **361**(9371):1767–1772).

Finding the responsible virus and defining the syndrome of SARS are just the beginning of a long and difficult journey, which we hope will culminate in the effective treatment and prevention of SARS. Along the way, we must find the necessary tools: rapid and sensitive diagnostic tests, effective and safe antiviral drugs, pragmatic and compliable infection control measures, and finally a safe and effective vaccine. All these will not come without painstaking research.

At present, our tools are rather unwieldy. The antibody test using the infected cell line as antigen only starts to become positive at around day 10, and it is only by the 28th day that most SARS cases would mount an antibody response. We are hoping that by cloning the viral genes in *Escherichia coli*, that this "bacterial factory" will manufacture recombinant viral proteins that can be used for the production of more sensitive and specific antibody tests.

As for the rapid RT-PCR, this test has returned positive for only 25 per cent of the SARS patients at the time of admission. It will need a lot of refinement to boost its sensitivity to above 90 per cent. This is becoming a reality after we have learned how to optimize the RNA extraction, choice of the primer sequence, testing condition, additional amplification step called nested reaction, and a final hybridization step.

The following are other challenges and difficulties that we will face on the way.

Our histopathological findings from the tissues of deceased SARS patients suggest that macrophages were a prominent cell in these tissues. Whether these were contributing to the lung pathology was a consideration to ponder.

Also, the viral load (density of viral presence) studies show that the virus increases in number during the first ten days and then decreases in number afterwards, irrespective of whether the patient is improving or deteriorating. This means that the patient may deteriorate even while the viral load is decreasing. For these reasons, we think that that at least part of the damage is directly related to the immune response of the host. This is the reason why steroids were included in our treatment: to dampen the so-called "excessive" immune response. This may, in turn, decrease lung damage and thus delay respiratory failure and the need for intubation in the intensive care unit.

However, such immunosuppressive treatment is associated with various potentially fatal side effects, which include bacterial or fungal super-infections (catching other diseases because of a weakened immune system).

The final answer to the treatment of SARS must lie in the development of an effective antiviral agent. If we can halt viral replication, we will also stop the excessive immune response. At this point in time, there is still no randomized placebo control trial to show whether any antivirals are effective with respect to the new coronavirus. Ribavirin, a classic broad-spectrum drug, by itself, does not appear to be effective. This was used during the early stages of the outbreak as an anti-viral agent when the causative pathogen was still unknown. Later, we continued to use relatively low doses of Ribavirin as an immunomodulator because this drug has been shown to be highly effective for this purpose in the treatment of fulminant hepatitis in mice caused by a mouse coronavirus. So an effective antiviral agent is yet to be found. Randomized placebo control clinical trials should be conducted to ascertain the effectiveness of the various antivirals showing activity in the test tube, to prepare for the eventuality of the epidemic returning in the coming winter.

The complete genomes of four different SARS coronavirus strains were completed by four different centers in Canada, the United States, and Hong Kong about a month after the discovery of the virus. From this we know of at least a number of enzymatic targets for antiviral therapy.[5] These include the RNA replicase (enzyme that replicate the viral genome); the proteases

---

[5] Viral DNA contains enzymes, or catalysts, that are vital for the life processes of a virus, for example, replication. During infection, the host cell is made to assist in the production of these enzymes, thus in effect helping the virus to replicate. Inhibiting the production of enzymes in the host cell will kill the virus.

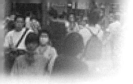

(enzymes that process the proteins so that they can be functional); and methyltransferase (enzymes that process the RNA). Researchers are now rushing to screen combinatorial chemical libraries (large stocks of compounds called "chemical backbones" with different modifications) to find an effective antiviral treatment for SARS.

Another line of attack is to disrupt some function of the virus itself. One of the most important surface targets for antiviral treatment is the Spike protein. This protein makes up the surface projections that give the virus the morphology (shape) of a crown. It functions like a claw which allows the virus to attach itself to human cells and draws the virus envelope to the human cell so that it fuses with the cell membrane. This fusion process allows the virus to enter the cell to start a new cycle of infection and multiplication from one virus to millions of viruses. To halt the fusion process, short chains of amino acids are designed to glue up the mechanical apparatus of this claw so that the virus can no longer invade the human cell. However, all these exciting new drugs now being fashioned in the laboratories will only go to the stage of human trial after at least one year and will not be commercially available until after two to three years. Countless experiments are needed, both in test tubes and animals, before a drug can be shown to be effective and safe enough to justify its trial on humans.

Similar difficulties apply in the development of a vaccine. The easiest way to obtain a vaccine is to kill the live virus with formalin so that it is not infectious but still retains its immunogenicity, i.e., the ability to stimulate a protective immune response from the human host. However this method sometimes brings about an immune response that, instead of being protective, leads to a much more severe reaction if and when the recipient contracts the live virus. This type of disaster has happened before when inactivated measles virus and respiratory syncytial virus were used as vaccines.

Vaccines can also be produced by simple sub-culturing of a virus under low temperature for a long time. Under such conditions, genetic mutations may accumulate in such a way that the virus can still multiply in humans, but harmlessly. This approach has been successfully used in the prevention of polio, measles, mumps and rubella. However, coronaviruses are well known for reshuffling their genome by recombination of large fragments of genetic material from different strains of the virus. Indeed new strains of pathogenic coronavirus resulting from recombination between the live vaccine and the

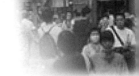

Where did this new coronavirus come from? Our genetic information already suggested that an animal source was the most likely possibility.

pathogenic wild virus has been discovered in poultry after the use of a live and weakened vaccine for the prevention of a chicken coronavirus infection. Thus the manipulation of live viruses for vaccines in the case of the coronavirus has to proceed, if at all, with much care.

Perhaps the safest way to develop the SARS coronavirus vaccine is the use of recombinant biotechnology. We can now fuse fragments of viral genes with very safe carriers such as adenovirus or vaccinia vectors, which cannot, or only briefly, multiply in human cells without any damaging effect. The safest way is to induce protective immune response by a recombinant viral protein produced by *Escherichia coli*, a common gut bacteria which acts as a factory for the production of viral protein after the viral gene is cloned into the bacteria.

It will be quite some time before we will have a candidate vaccine that is shown to be effective in protecting monkeys from the artificial inoculation with SARS coronavirus. This will then take another epidemic before we can test the vaccine in field trials. Of course nobody in his right mind would welcome this opportunity.

Before we have a good vaccine, the only preventive strategy for SARS is the diligent and appropriate use of quarantine and other infection control measures. Dr. Wing-hong Seto, the consultant microbiologist in Queen Mary Hospital, the teaching hospital affiliated to the University of Hong Kong, has clearly demonstrated that the consistent and proper use of masks and hand washing are highly effective in the prevention of SARS among hospital staff. Lapses in these simple preventive measures or protection that is overdone (such as use of heavy, clumsy, double or triple protective clothing that may result in the wearer making mistakes or lapses) can be associated with hospital acquired SARS.

Where did this new coronavirus come from? Our genetic information already suggested that an animal source was the most likely possibility. In our

The first-hand collection of data on emerging infectious diseases should become a perpetual concern and part of our overall healthcare program.

collaboration with the Shenzheng CDC, Dr. Guan Yi and Dr. Zheng Bo-jian from our department demonstrated that the SARS coronavirus can be found in the excreta of many civet cats and a few other wild animals caught for preparing game food. They also showed that sera from those people working closely with such animals had a high prevalence of antibody against this SARS coronavirus. The SARS virus may well be a zoonosis (an infectious disease transmitted from vertebrates to human). The virus might have repeatedly jumped to humans without being detected because it had never mutated sufficiently to cause human-to-human spread. These series of mutations might have sufficiently changed the property of the virus so as to almost cause a pandemic.

Hong Kong has much to learn from this major epidemic that has affected over 1700 people and killed almost 300. Known infectious diseases are less perilous because we understand how they behave. SARS, being an emerging infectious disease, was virtually an unknown entity.

The first lesson to remember is how difficult it was for us to fight an enemy we know very little about. So we should make every effort to obtain intelligence on any uncommon diseases in China, or even in other parts of the world, as soon as they surface. Our public health authorities should attach field officers to investigative teams in China or elsewhere, and first-hand information can be relayed home through the web. In this way, data can be analyzed and strategies formulated, hopefully, even before an epidemic hits Hong Kong.

Such an approach requires a fundamental change in mind-set. We confront a disease not when it hits us but before it hits us. The first-hand collection of data on emerging infectious diseases should become a perpetual concern and part of our overall healthcare program.

Another important element in this approach is the honing of skills and maintenance of vigilance. This is analogous to the earthquake rescue teams that exist in many countries. Since major earthquakes are quite rare, many such teams participate in rescue efforts wherever they occur. Thus they are continually tested in real-life contexts, which helps to keep both skills and knowledge at optimal levels. Medical teams can do the same.

Hong Kong and southern China, where large populations of both humans and animals live in close proximity, are prime settings for infectious diseases and even bio-terrorism. Developing both the expertise and infrastructure for intercepting, or at least preparing for, diseases before they cross our borders would prove invaluable.

The second lesson concerns the part played by wet markets and hospitals as "epidemic centers" (epi-centers) or amplification premises in the SARS outbreak, and perhaps as potential epidemic centers for other infectious diseases. Information released by the Guangdong CDC (Centre for Disease Control) suggested that the first SARS patients had clear histories of contact with wild game food animals and their risk of contracting SARS seems to be related to proximity to wet markets. This reminds me of the 1997 outbreak of influenza in Hong Kong. The lesson is that unless carefully managed, places like markets and hospitals can potentially be settings where pathogens concentrate and multiply in either animals or human.

The running of wet markets in Hong Kong should be thoroughly reviewed. Premises where shoppers might become carriers or victims of zoonotic microbes through contact with animal excreta should be a thing of the past. The upgrading of all wets markets should be a critical and integral part of Hong Kong's effort to become a modern and clean city.

The SARS outbreak highlighted the failure of infection control in many hospitals. Massive outbreaks started in hospitals and then spilled out into the community. A single infected patient returning home gave rise to a type of SARS outbreak at Amoy Gardens (an apartment complex) that was

The lesson is that unless carefully managed, places like markets and hospitals can potentially be settings where pathogens concentrate and multiply in either animals or human.

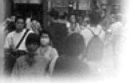

unprecedented in our history. Thus, the disaster that might have been avoided, if hospital infection control and the flow of information had been more effective.

The lesson here is that hospitals can be the "Normandy-beaches" for future epidemics to land on, or premises where infectious microbes may gain a foothold in our city. Accordingly, meticulous infection control must become part of the hospital culture and rooted in the mindset of all healthcare workers. A detailed investigation into the administration, infection control processes (such as the requirements for closure of wards), architectural design of hospital wards, and personnel training should be undertaken. Lapses at all levels should be identified and corrected.

Risk assessment should be done for every patient admitted to emergency rooms or clinics, with a scoring system that streams patients either to single-room isolation, or a multi-bed cohort, or a general ward for observation.

Real time surveillance of hospital staff illnesses such as fever, respiratory illness, diarrhea, exanthematous illnesses through obligatory reporting of all suspected infections, which may or may not require sick leave, should be implemented in all hospitals. This should be the most sensitive parameter for auditing infection control, and an important early warning signal for hospital outbreaks of SARS-like illnesses.

The number of beds should be decreased to allow infection control measures to be properly implemented. In many wards, the beds are so close together that patients can touch the next bed simply by stretching out an arm.

Lectures on and practices of infection control are largely ignored among medical undergraduates and student nurses. Hand hygiene and other isolation procedures are seldom fully complied with. Thus common antibiotic resistant agent such as MRSA (methicillin resistant *Staphylococcus aureus*) are rapidly disseminating in hospitals. MRSA can also spread by contact and occasionally by respiratory droplets like SARS. If hospitals cannot control MRSA, it is unlikely that SARS can be controlled if it returns.

Building a culture of absolute compliance with infection control measures should be a top priority: a matter of life and death. This message should be somehow repeated religiously to every healthcare worker daily at the start of every shift. There is always a chance that one of our patients is going to be the index patient of the next outbreak. One never knows.

Nobody knows whether SARS will return. We should definitely prepare for a possible comeback in the winter because most respiratory viruses have shown seasonality.

The third lesson is the importance of effective communication to both healthcare workers and the public. When an outbreak affects a large number of healthcare workers, many doctors and nurses will be caring for their colleagues and personal friends. The recent outbreak demonstrated that this could be a source of deep emotional distress, which in turn has important repercussions on the public's perception of the outbreak.

When highly stressed hospital personnel are interviewed by the media, they often respond emotionally rather than objectively. Stressful responses tend to be slanted, erratic, and even inaccurate. This can seriously undermine the credibility of those in authority. Unless coherent and authoritative information is continually forthcoming during an outbreak, public confidence can dissipate. If, added to these, the public senses that the disease is getting an upper hand and sees more healthcare workers stricken, panic may ensue. We came very close to this in Hong Kong.

This situation may be avoided by setting up independent emergency medical teams, which are sent to wherever a relatively large number of hospital staff are being infected. Such teams of experts can bring objectivity and stability, and work to defuse highly emotional and stressful situations.

Their jobs might include assisting hospital staff to take stock of and control their situation, as well as making sure that information is disseminated to the public in a cohesive and accurate manner.

Nobody knows whether SARS will return. We should definitely prepare for a possible comeback in the winter because most respiratory viruses have shown seasonality. We have no reason to believe that this virus would be different. Indeed the two previously known human coronaviruses tend to cause outbreaks during the late winter and early spring. This time round, the first case in Guangdong happened in November, the epidemic peaked in February, then disappeared by April.

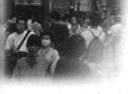

A final lesson is that microbes far outnumber the human population and their capability to undergo genetic mutation outruns mankind's ability to entirely control them. We can only continue with diligent preparations and surveillance, and do our best to minimize the damage as a result of their occasional rampages.

Acknowledgements

We thank Dr Seto Wing Luk (PhD in communication) for his help in reading the manuscript and making helpful suggestions. Our thanks also to Ms Sook-Cheng Lim of World Scientific Publishing for her interest and support.

KWOK-YUNG YUEN

Dr. Kwok-yung Yuen is Professor and Head, Department of Microbiology, The University of Hong Kong. Prof. Yuen started his career as a medical doctor (MBBS, HKU) in 1981, going on to become a surgeon (Fellow of the Royal College of Surgeons, UK) in 1986. He has worked as a medical microbiologist since 1992. He is the academic director of the postgraduate diploma course of infectious disease (HKU). Prof. Yuen devotes half of his time to seeing patients and half to research and teaching. He is thus able to use the scientific findings gained through research of the medical problems encountered during clinical practice to directly benefit his patients.

Dr. Yuen's area of interest is focused on emerging infectious disease of regional importance. He has been a leader of infectious disease traninig of both clinical microbiologists and physicians for the last 15 years.

Dr. Yuen and his research team at The University of Hong Kong discovered the agent that caused the Severe Acute Respiratory Syndrome in Hong Kong in 2003. This novel coronavirus is now recognized by the WHO as the primary cause of SARS. Their team is the third in the world to complete the sequencing of the genome of the virus.

In 1977, Prof. Yuen's team developed rapid tests for avian flu A H5N1. He was invited by the government to serve in the Advisory Council on Food and Environmental Hygiene, Environmental and Food Bureau and the Expert Working Group on Avian Influenza, Dept of Health.

Dr. Yuen's other significant contributions to research include development of the first serological tests for rapid diagnosis of the serious fungal infection caused by *Penicillin marneffei* and institution of a surveillance program to eliminate platelet transfusion bacteremia.

Dr. Yuen has published over 200 papers which are cited by PubMed. Several of the papers were published in the prestigious journal *Lancet*.

Correspondence to: Prof. K.Y. Yuen, E-mail: kyyuen@hkucc.hku.hk

Malik Peiris

Dr. JSM Peiris, MBBS, D Phil (Oxcon) is Professor at the Department of Microbiology, The University of Hong Kong. His research interests are:

- Influenza: ecology, epidemiology, evolution and pathogenesis of animal and human influenza, disease burden of human influenza, new diagnostic methods.
- Human herpesvirus 6 (HHV-6) and 7 (HHV-7).
- Virus-macrophage interactions and pathogenesis.
- Clinical virology: diagnostic methods and clinical management.

Current Research Interests:

- SARS: aetiology, pathogenesis, diagnosis, antivirals, vaccines
- Influenza: ecology, epidemiology, evolution and pathogenesis of animal and human influenza (see influenza research group), disease burden of human influenza, new diagnostic methods.
- Virus-macrophage interactions and pathogenesis.
- Clinical virology: diagnostic methods and clinical management.

International Recognition (selected examples):

a) Invited Plenary Lectures and chair sessions at International meetings (e.g. National Institutes of Allergy and Infectious Diseases, SARS: Developing a Research Response, May 30, 2003; WHO Global Conference on Severe Acute Respiratory Syndrome (SARS): where do we go from here? June 17/18 2003.

b) Temporary Advisor to WHO on Global Influenza Program; SARS aetiology & epidemiology.

c) Associate editor, Journal of Clinical Virology.

d) Member of a "WHO Informal Consultation on Research on the molecular biology and epidemiology of animal and human viruses in Asia", May 2000 and invited to be an instructor at "WHO Training Course on Animal Influenza Surveillance". National Veterinary Research Institute Harbin, China, May 2001.

e) Contribute chapters to prestigious and "standard" books in the field, including The Oxford Textbook of Medicine, Manson's Tropical Diseases and the Encyclopaedia of Arthropod-transmitted infections of Man and Domesticated Animals.

Section IV

Singapore

11

Sars, Policy-making and Lesson-drawing

by KHAI LEONG HO

Introduction

The reactions of Asian governments to the crisis of the Severe Acute Respiratory Syndrome (SARS) epidemic are lessons of policy-making and policy implementation par excellence. Countries affected by this new viral outbreak, such as China, Hong Kong, Vietnam, Singapore, Malaysia and Taiwan, have been compiling and implementing various urgent measures and sustained efforts to deal with the problem. The political, legal and cultural contexts of these countries have certainly influenced the ways in which these governments reacted to the crisis. As is evident from the respective histories of especially their public health sectors, the reactions of these governments have emerged as useful explanatory variables in reflecting upon policy actions and inactions.

The repercussions for the Asian countries in the face of the outbreak will certainly resonate well beyond the loss of life and economic losses, for social

> **Some governments, like China have received very poor ratings, whereas others, like Singapore, have attracted a slew of very positive comments from even its most skeptical foreign critics.**

consequences will be equally severe, as has been attested by the social and political unrests in China's hard-to-reach countryside. However, the long-term consequences of these repercussions have yet to be determined. At present, the situation is further heightened by the fact that the various Asian governments' actions and inactions, attitudes and postures, responses and reactions are constantly the subjects of scrutiny by the international community, who are concerned with both the economic and political consequences of this crisis. Indeed, it is true that the extent to which the world views these Asian governments and their abilities to deal with the contagious disease will invariably determine the political and economic future of the governments in power.

The assessments so far have been mixed. Some governments, like China have received very poor ratings, whereas others, like Singapore, have attracted a slew of very positive comments from even its most skeptical foreign critics. Despite the differences in evaluation outcomes, these countries ultimately realized that effective settlement of the problem implies an inherent need for mutual cooperation, collaboration and learning so that this serious public health crisis can be ameliorated.

The discussions here will focus on the different phases of the various governments' reactions to the crisis, followed by an attempt to explicate the policy lessons that have been and could be learnt from this devastating experience.

Different Phases of Governments' Reactions

Very often, when a focusing event and crisis is without any modern precedence, governments (being bureaucracies not known for its thinking abilities) tend to be taken aback. The initial period of "freezing" — being held up, so to speak, can range from "short" (a few hours) to "medium" (a few days or weeks) to "long" (a few months). The moment this "freezing" period comes to an end, the realization that the problem is indeed a serious one ultimately dawns upon them, resulting in the dramatic alteration from initial panic to a somber hunt for solutions.

SARS, with its ability to bring about rapid, unexpected fatalities and economic paralysis, threw Asian governments off guard. Although such widespread viral infections are not new in these modern times, the speed at which SARS spreads and causes fatal death certainly brings much alarm to modern Asian governments with very faint memories of viral infections in their histories. Although this may not be so much the case in China or Malaysia, it does little in terms of enervating the fear of the epidemic.

From the public policy perspective, Asian governments' reactions can be divided into five distinct phrases.

1. *Cover-up/Hiding of Information*

News reports have suggested that the SARS virus most certainly originated from China. As such, in retrospect, the Chinese government's handling of the outbreak constituted a critical phase of the development of the crisis. While there is some truth in the accusation by Taiwanese politicians and officials that if China had revealed the problem to the rest of the world on time, the severity of the crisis could have been significantly reduced, the reality is that the Chinese government, both provincial and central, did not deal with the problem decisively.

News of falsified communications, deliberate misinformation, obstruction of United Nations assessment teams and reluctance to reveal the full extent of the epidemic to the World Health Organization in different ways, were strategies adopted to mislead and conceal.

The problem was further aggravated by the fact that Chinese government officials covered up the severity and spread of the disease. News of falsified communications, deliberate misinformation, obstruction of United Nations assessment teams and reluctance to reveal the full extent of the epidemic to the World Health Organization in different ways, were strategies adopted to mislead and conceal. To the chagrin of the international community, Chinese officials later admitted to this foolish and irresponsible activity. As could be anticipated, heads rolled and lower ranking officials were made scapegoats in a political game commonplace in China.

2. Governments' Knee-jerk Reactions to the Problem and Fear among the Public

Given that SARS is a new disease, public officials were unacquainted as to how they should react to the problem. Most of the time, reactions, if any, were ad-hoc decisions aimed to counter criticisms. For instance, the Hong Kong government wasted precious time in containing the disease only to realize that its limited measures were ineffective when the residents in Amoy Gardens became infected. It then scrambled to assure the world that things were under control, when the number of infected cases continued to rise.

While China was belatedly waking up to a crisis, Taiwan, which had had time to prepare for the worse, slacked in its effort to do so. The decision to close and quarantine the staff, patients and visitors at Hoping Hospital in Taipei was done so hurriedly that few were willing to accept the consequences that followed. The public, without much information, began to panic, subsequently suggesting that the knee-jerk reactions by the Taipei city government aided in the spread of suspicions and alarm among the public.

3. Knowing more about the Disease, Grouping Together to find Solution

As events progressed, governments gradually came to know more about the virus and how it spread. Measures such as quarantines, temperature taking, etc., were instituted. Vietnam and Singapore took the lead in many of these

> **Singapore's authoritarian political context, its physical size, and quick responses were all cited as the right steps in the right directions.**

measures. These countries were particularly successful due to the structure of laws that they had inherited from the French and British systems; this in turn enabled the governments to act fairly quickly to quarantine those who were in contact with SARS infected patients. The Singapore legislature, known for its swift passing of laws, met quickly to legislate harsher penalties for those who defied the quarantine laws.

Scientists everywhere began to scramble to find a cure for the virus, only to realize that such a cure would take a few more years to materialize. Therefore, all the "breakthroughs" and "discoveries", supposedly conducted by the scientific communities as reported by the news media, were mostly premature.

4. Learning from What Other Countries have done

When the crisis dragged on into a month without any signs of abating, many governments began to see the inadequacies of their measures. Thus, they began to look elsewhere for more effective solutions and measures. An illustration of this is Taiwan's constant reference to Singapore's effective policies in containing the disease. Singapore's authoritarian political context, its physical size, and quick responses were all cited as the right steps in the right directions.

A fine example is the use of temperature scanners which Singaporean companies claim to have first developed and produced. Using thermal imaging sensor technologies, the system unobtrusively measures the temperatures of people. Furthermore, this new Infrared Fever Sensing System camera is able to help identify people with fevers arriving from SARS-hit countries. It was first used in Singapore's Changi International Airport, and very quickly came to be installed in the country's land checkpoints as well. Likewise, Hong Kong, Malaysia and China also acquired the equipment to check inbound and outbound passengers.

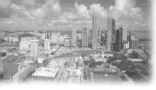

5. Settling to Combat a Long-term Crisis

The SARS crisis has finally prompted many governments to reflect on a long-term solution to the problem. With the exposure of the inadequacies of the public healthcare system, standards of hygiene, and failures of legislation, the government began a campaign of public education on hygienic practices, thereby establishing the major emphasis of public policy in the months ahead. "Living with SARS" already has become a slogan which many governments are using in their public drive to raise awareness.

It is apparent that the SARS crisis has tested the governments' ability to solve problems in an effective matter. These responses went through stages: fear, secrecy, panic in the search for solutions, and ultimately mutual cooperation in a bid to resolve a major crisis.

Lessons Learnt

The SARS crisis clearly shows that a major focusing event is able to significantly alter the contours of governments' policy-making. In particular, the post-event developments have highlighted a few lessons learnt.

The first and most pertinent lesson learnt is that governmental transparency in all its actions is of the utmost importance. Given that transparency is a generic term that includes honestly reporting and releasing of information, such an open state of policy-making will benefit everybody in the long run. This is as opposed to a closed system that will inevitably generate fear and uncertainties, which serves only to breed rumors and apprehensions about the state of affairs. The Asian financial crisis in 1997 to a great extent was a result of the secretive nature of financial dealings and policy-making.

The problem with the current epidemic was due to the improper compilation and analysis of SARS numbers. It is difficult to fathom the intentions of governments' persisting in treating the SARS outbreak as a "state secret", for regarding public health as a "state secret" is similar to an individual's inability or denial of his state of health. In this global age, governments should realize that concealing information can only warrant disastrous results. Global travels and cross-border transfers, have made the world much smaller. As a result, citizens, regional and international communities alike have been equally vocal in their demands for transparency in government decision-making. The current SARS outbreak shows how an increasingly interconnected world is changing the way diseases are being perceived and spread.

The Chinese government has been accused of initially concealing important information. The fact that the Chinese government did not share the information earlier with the public and healthcare workers aggravated the problem. The actual number of cases were not honestly reported, thus rendering the situation worse. Indeed, the Chinese government's initial cover-up says a lot about the authoritarian nature of its political system.

China's less than open approach to information is consistent with her past behaviors. The continuing lack of transparency in China reflects the ways in which she conducts her business, both locally and globally. At a time when China desperately requires foreign investment and tourist dollars for her ever increasing appetite of economic development, the withholding of information about SARS cases certainly hampered her credibility as ambiguity and uncertainty are not condoned by international businesses.

The initial response of the Malaysian government was also criticized by many observers. It was reported that its first response to the crisis was to send a letter to newspaper editors to tone down any reporting of SARS cases. Later, reporters were discouraged from visiting victims, due to the social stigmatization that may be brought to their families. Such actions were unsurprising, given that Malaysians were amused by the government's

The first and most pertinent lesson learnt is that governmental transparency in all its actions is of the utmost importance. Given that transparency is a generic term that includes honestly reporting and releasing of information, such an open state of policy-making will benefit everybody in the long run.

> **The second lesson that countries can learn from the crisis is that coordination of policy is of paramount importance. Coordination between departments/ministries/level of the government within a country; and coordination between countries.**

continued ban on the publication of air-quality ratings for fear of "deterring" tourists. Rumors in the country began to emerge and the credibility of the Barisan Nasional government officials was lessened.

Indeed, if countries were to succeed in their social, political and economic transformations and their integration into the global mainstream, transparency and clarity in handling of problems must be the first prerequisite. While it is taken for granted that the interests of a sovereign state should always be protected, information that could potentially have significant impact on the fate of other countries should be disclosed honestly and expediently.

The second lesson that countries can learn from the crisis is that coordination of policy is of paramount importance. In this case, there are two levels of coordination: Coordination between departments/ministries/level of the government within a country; and coordination between countries.

The first level of coordination was apparently most difficult given the fact that many governments were caught off guard. The chaotic state of affairs was mostly apparent in Hong Kong and Taiwan. In Singapore, an inter-ministerial committee was formed in order to avoid any delays or holdups in making decisions. Coordination certainly needs to be improved in order for the players involved to arrive at a concerted effort in combating the disease.

The second level of coordination was not well executed either. The mysterious nature of the disease and the rising death toll, led many governments to adopt several myopic ad-hoc decisions. These ad hoc decisions implemented in a futile bid to protect their borders were quickly lifted when it was deemed illogical. Instead of solving the problem, banning their citizens from traveling to other countries, for example, only resulted in more confusion. The apparent lack of concerted international cooperation has hindered common efforts to stop the spread of the epidemic. However, it should be noted that under WHO guidelines and with the help of countries in North America, Europe and Asia, scientists were able to identify the SARS virus in less than four weeks.

The third lesson learnt is that communities as well as governments should avoid excessive politicization when dealing with a crisis. Of course, politics may not be altogether avoidable, but still, it needs to be minimized in order for the derivation of a quick decision. Upon the occurrence of the crisis, effective management rather than the democratic process of decision-making should be of the utmost concern. Politicizing by political opponents and factional rivals would only serve to further aggravate the problem.

In this regard, the Taiwanese political polity has demonstrated to the world that it is a negative example of bad politics holding sway over effective management. Politicians were too caught up in accusing their oppositions as well as the Communist government in mainland China in spreading the disease. Or to quote the words of its former Health Minister Twu Shiing-jer, "After hiding the epidemic for over four months, Beijing still failed to deal with the SARS virus." This clearly shows that politicians and officials were distracted from the obvious — namely, the expedient need to tackle the problem professionally.

The rest of the world, however, has not fared any better. The ASEAN meeting in Bangkok on 29 April, with China, Japan and South Korea, pointedly omitted Taiwan amongst its discussants. For six years, the World Health Organization (WHO) has refused to admit Taiwan as a member or even as an observer in deference to mainland China's opposing claim that healthcare in Taiwan is its responsibility. The spread of SARS to Taiwan has shown the absurdity of excluding 23 million Taiwanese outside the world's health community. It is a pity that politics has again reared its ugly head in a matter that is strictly concerned with health and human life.

The fourth lesson learnt is that problem definition is a crucial stage in policy-making. Granted then that this is a legitimate problem, how and when do governments decide if this is a problem? What category does the problem fall under? Is this a "pressing" problem which actively intrudes upon the policy agenda, or a "chosen" problem, one which policymakers can wait? Obviously, as was evident in the case of China, the situation was not deemed a pressing one by the government; rather, it was deemed as merely another condition that it has been used to handling. As a result of this confidence, no viable

> **After an initial period of uncertainty and hesitation, Singapore's government very quickly defined this as a problem as serious as that of terrorism and war, and thus, immediately called for the setting up a ministerial committee to combat the problem.**

solutions were conceptualized to tackle the problem. Some governments, however, have characterized the combating of the disease as a war. After an initial period of uncertainty and hesitation, Singapore's government very quickly defined this as a problem as serious as that of terrorism and war, and thus, immediately called for the setting up a ministerial committee to combat the problem. Policy-makers, therefore, must have a sense of urgency and crisis. If the pressure and exigency are not present, it is unlikely that the bureaucracy would commit all its resources to deal with the problem.

The fifth lesson is one of sustaining an effective policy. It has to be understood that in order for the effective long-term sustenance of any policy, public education is imperative. This campaign, however, needs to be implemented concomitant with a genuine gesture of a government's transparency. If government has no legitimacy, it is unlikely that the public will feel an obligation to obey and take the necessary precautions to safeguard public health. This in turn renders it more difficult for public education and public campaigns to penetrate the countryside compared with the cities. Chinese premier Wen Jiabao has already warned that the situation would be worse if the outbreak spills from the cities to the countryside, where the majority of China's 1.3 billion people live with minimal healthcare.

The sixth lesson learnt is this: In a crisis situation, individual privacy and liberty may have to be sacrificed for the sake of public interest. The perennial debate in public policy is whether personal freedom is necessarily a victim of community interest. In cases of quarantine, policies inevitably invaded one's freedom and privacy. Even the act of temperature taking itself is an act that intrudes on personal freedom. Indeed, increased personal freedom is one of

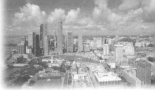

the cherished byproducts of the last two decades of economic reforms. Until any real impending threat to their lives is felt, most people tend to just ignore the government's plea in their continued belief that the campaigns are little more than ritualistic routines.

Inept Policies Leading to Political Legitimacy and Crisis

A connection must be drawn between inept policies and political legitimacy of a government. Let us take the case of China where the political impacts of SARS are most obvious. Apart from widespread fear of contracting the disease, there was mounting popular disgust over the perceived laxness and lies on the part of the authorities. This sparked a series of violent incidents in the countryside like the riots that broke out in the eastern Zhejiang province, in protest against a decision by the local authorities to provide temporary accommodation for eight villagers returning home from a SARS-infected area.

China's new political leadership was under tremendous pressure to demonstrate to the world at large that it was different from the old guards in terms of style and substance. After weeks of international pressure, the Chinese government of President and Communist Party leader Hu Jintao and Prime Minister Wen Jiabao fired two prominent officials for failing to address the threat posed by SARS. This action was perhaps one step too late because there were already warning signs of a major economic disruption within the country and the rest of the Asia-Pacific region.

While the SARS crisis may serve as a challenge that would enhance the legitimacy of political leadership for some governments, it simultaneously may also eventually bring down ineffective public managers and political leaders. The governments have little time to lose: failure to act decisively could mutate the SARS health crisis into a political and social time bomb. As we have seen thus far, the SARS crisis has had huge political implications for China and the rest of the world. Depending on how the crisis progresses, it may either trigger a political crisis or serve as the catalyst for further reform. The call for reforms will have to come not only from the public, but also from the factions within governments. After all, it should be borne in mind that should citizens observe no improvement in their lots despite making explicit their demands to governments, the legitimacy of the government becomes doubtful.

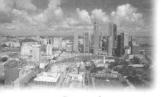

Conclusions

The considerable dissatisfaction and unhappiness with policy reactions thus far has only succeeded in intensifying the search for definitive answers and effective solutions. One might reasonably expect that the tone of the next phrase of governments' discourse delivered in response to a focusing event will be more reconciliatory than combative. This is evident from the fact that though the outbreak has been "effectively contained," the governments are still urging continued vigilance by citizens and healthcare workers.

Fighting the SARS epidemic is akin to fighting a war, perhaps not unlike that of anti-terrorism; governments need to be vigilant at all times. In addition, this public health problem also requires politicians to move away from politicking. This crisis has rendered governments a much needed wake-up call, informing them of the merits of committing all manner of resources, professional, economic and political, to halt the outbreak. At present, after the initial period of panic, fear and scarcity of information on the disease, governments as well as people have come to the defining phase in combating the disease: (1) the scientific community and medical profession have to find a cure within a reasonable period; (2) governments have to tighten policy measures to contain the disease and to educate the public; and (3) the people have to act responsibly both personally and communally to perhaps act as checks on the governments' inactions.

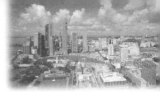

KHAI LEONG HO

Dr. Khai Leong Ho (Ph.D. Ohio State, 1988) is a researcher at the Institute of Southeast Asian Studies, Singapore. He has taught at the Public Policy Programme, National University of Singapore and Department of Political Science, West Virginia University, and was a visiting fellow at the Japan Institute of International Affairs, Tokyo, Japan. He was appointed as a member of the international network and panel of assessors for grant applications, the Program on Global Security and Cooperation (GSC), Social Science Research Council, Washington, D.C., U.S.A. (2001–2002). His current research interests include Malaysia and Singapore politics, corporate governance, administrative reforms, and public policy initiatives. His publications have appeared in *The Journal of Comparative Asian Development, The Pacific Review, Asian Survey, Asian Journal of Public Administration, Pacific Focus, Asian Journal of Political Science, Internationales Asienforum (International Quarterly for Asian Studies), Journal of Contemporary China, Southeast Asian Affairs,* and *Asian Perspective.* His latest publications are *The Politics of Policy-making in Singapore* (Singapore: Oxford University Press, 2000) (the new edition will be published as *Shared Responsibilities, Unshared Power. The Politics of Policy-making* in 2003 by Eastern Universities Press) and *Performance and Crisis of Governance of Mahathir's Administration* (co-editor) (Singapore: Times Academic Press, 2001). (This book has been translated into Malay, entitled *Pentabiran Mahathir. Prestasi dan Krisis dalam Pemerintahan,* Singapore: Times Books International, 2003).

Correspondence to: Dr. Khai Leong Ho, E-mail: polhokl@nus.edu.sg.

12

SARS: A Psychological Perspective

by *GEORGE D. BISHOP*

1. Introduction

There can be no doubt but that SARS has had a tremendous impact, both psychologically and behaviorally. Even though SARS is a medical condition and much of the effort to understand and contain SARS has been medical in nature, it is clear that the psychological impact of SARS has been far out of proportion to the number of people who have actually contracted the disease. As of mid–July, there had been roughly 8,500 probable cases of SARS, most of them in China, with a confirmed death toll of just over 800. In Singapore the number of cases stood at 238 with 33 people dead. In absolute terms these are small numbers. However, SARS has resulted in substantial behavioral change as well as a great deal of fear and has had a devastating effect on the economies of affected countries.

In many respects, the fear and behavioral changes are quite understandable. Given its seemingly sudden appearance as well as the uncertainty surrounding

> **People respond in terms of how they understand the disease on an intellectual level and also the emotions evoked by the disease. These processes are closely interrelated and occur simultaneously but are separate and have distinct implications.**

the disease, its spread and mortality are guaranteed to raise alarm. The fact that it appears to be spread through simple social contact with an infected person also heightens the fear. However, it is also important to keep SARS in perspective and, while taking precautions, find ways of going about our normal activities. In reality the number of people who have contracted SARS is small. For example, some 1,800 Singaporeans have been diagnosed with HIV since the first case was detected in 1985, roughly 7.5 times the number of people contracting SARS. Further, the fatality rate of SARS pales in comparison with AIDS, where the rate is considered to be close to 100%. The mortality rate for SARS is also lower than dengue fever which claims 20% of its victims. This is not to downplay the seriousness of SARS but rather to place it in a larger context.

2. Responding to SARS Psychologically

From research on how the general public deals with illness and illness threats, we know that responses to illness threats take place on two levels, the cognitive and the emotional. People respond in terms of how they understand the disease on an intellectual level and also the emotions evoked by the disease. These processes are closely interrelated and occur simultaneously but are separate and have distinct implications. Understanding psychological responses to SARS requires that we address both of these.

Perhaps the most difficult aspect of SARS to deal with has been its uncertainty and the speed of its appearance. SARS erupted on the scene very rapidly and seemingly without warning. Although there had been cases in

China since November 2002, these first came to the world's attention in February 2003 with cases beginning to show up in Hong Kong and Vietnam at the end of February and in Singapore and Canada in March. The rapid increase in number of cases as well as its lightening spread between countries and the unknown cause was the source of great alarm. WHO issued travel advisories to airlines since the speed of spread between countries seemed to be facilitated by air travel and advised travelers to avoid infected areas.

Simultaneously, there was considerable confusion about the causes and about how the disease was spread. Scientists scrambled to identify the cause of the new condition and by the end of March, WHO announced that SARS appeared to be caused by a previously unknown strain of coronavirus, the family of viruses that causes the common cold. Because it appeared that the virus could spread very easily from an infected person, thousands of people believed possibly exposed to the virus were placed in quarantine in China, Hong Kong, Singapore and Toronto. Further, schools were closed and additional warnings were issued for travelers to avoid infected areas.

Couple this kind of uncertainty with a deadly virus and you have a perfect recipe for fear and, at times, panic. News reports indicated panic in China where, by some reports, residents were fleeing the city over their concern about SARS. With the WHO travel advisories, travels to Hong Kong, Singapore, China and Toronto took a nosedive, as travelers either chose other destinations or avoided traveling altogether. There were also reports of blatant discrimination against people perceived to be from a SARS affected area and some schools in the US stated explicitly that students coming from SARS affected areas were not welcome.

A. Worry about SARS

It is little wonder that responses to a worldwide online survey concerning beliefs among the lay public about SARS done by the author and a group of behavioral scientists known as the SARS Psychosocial Research Consortium showed that, on average, those living in both affected and unaffected areas were highly worried about SARS as a health problem, and those in affected areas in particular were worried about SARS in their region and of getting SARS themselves. Even those in unaffected areas reported some concern about

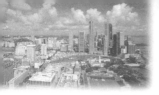

getting SARS, although their level of worry was somewhat below that for those in affected areas.

When we looked more closely at those worries, it was clear that they were closely associated with beliefs about SARS as a disease as well as behavioral responses to SARS and how people coped with the SARS threat. To get an idea of how people perceived SARS as a disease, those responding to the survey were asked about their beliefs about how SARS is spread, the seriousness of the SARS threat in various countries and also who they thought was at most risk of getting SARS. Worry about SARS was positively related to these beliefs, demonstrating very clearly the relationship between the cognitive and emotional response to this epidemic. People who indicated that they believed that SARS was very likely spread through various means, such as being near someone with SARS, through poor sanitation or poor personal hygiene, through sewage, cockroaches and even some ways in which SARS is not spread, such as by mosquitoes, also indicated more worry about getting SARS and about SARS in their region. Further, worry about SARS was related to beliefs that particular people, such as airline personnel, healthcare workers, or family or friends of SARS patients, were at particularly high risk of getting SARS. Also seeing the risk of SARS as being high in specific countries was related to higher levels of worry, regardless of whether the particular country had been identified by authorities as SARS-infected. For example, a number of respondents perceived a high risk of SARS in Malaysia and Japan even though these countries had very few cases and were never identified by WHO as SARS infected. There was a particularly strong relationship between beliefs about the seriousness of SARS in one's own country and worry, again regardless

People who indicated that they believed that SARS was very likely spread through various means, such as being near someone with SARS, through poor sanitation or poor personal hygiene... also indicated more worry about getting SARS and about SARS in their region.

of whether the country was SARS-affected. While many of the beliefs that people have about SARS may be accurate, others are not and it does not appear that the accuracy of the beliefs is the determining factor in their worry. Rather, it is simply the beliefs themselves that seem to be important as sources of worry.

It is important to note that worries are not, in themselves, necessarily bad. As long as they are not overly exaggerated they can play an important role in motivating people to remain vigilant. And, indeed, it appears that the worries about SARS were not overly exaggerated. To get an idea of the extent to which worries about SARS were exaggerated, we asked people to rate the likelihood of several undesirable events, including getting and dying from SARS as well as dying in a traffic accident, getting "the flu", getting cancer, and having a heart attack. People were quite accurate in stating that they were much less likely to get SARS or die from it than to get "the flu" or cancer or have a heart attack or have an accident at home. They did rate the likelihood of getting SARS as being higher than getting HIV, however, despite the fact that HIV has actually infected several times the number of Singaporeans than have been infected by SARS. On the whole, however, the level of concern about SARS appeared to be fairly well based in reality.

B. *Taking precautions*

With no cure available for SARS, the primary key to controlling the epidemic lies in getting people to take precautions. Respondents in our survey were asked to indicate which of a number of precautions they had taken to avoid getting SARS, including avoiding such activities as travel to SARS infected areas, eating in restaurants, shaking hands and travel in taxies as well as positive behaviors such as wearing a mask, washing hands and using disinfectants. Their answers showed that those in SARS affected areas were taking appropriate precautions with more than 80% indicating that they had washed their hands more often and nearly three quarters indicating that they had avoided travel to other SARS affected areas or had worn a mask. Those responding to the survey were also asked about steps they had taken to determine if they might have SARS, including taking one's temperature, going to the doctor, and paying close attention to the various possible SARS related

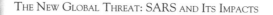

> **Their answers showed that those in SARS affected areas were taking appropriate precautions with more than 80% indicating that they had washed their hands more often and nearly three quarters indicating that they had avoided travel to other SARS affected areas or had worn a mask.**

symptoms. Taking one's temperature was the most commonly reported measure for detecting possible SARS, with over 80% of those in SARS affected areas indicating that they had done that. This is to be expected since a fever of about 38°C has been identified as the most reliable indicator of possible SARS.

As we would expect, concerns about SARS were related to the person's likelihood of taking precautions as well as taking steps to see if one might have SARS. Worry about getting SARS or dying from it was very strongly and positively related to the number of precautions taken regardless of whether respondents were from affected or unaffected areas. Interestingly, worry about SARS was related to actions taken to determine if the person had SARS, but only in unaffected areas. Compared with the unaffected areas, people in affected areas on average took more actions to detect possible SARS but the number of actions was not related to worry. Perhaps the strong encouragement of governments, employers and others in the affected areas to take such steps may have overridden individual worry as a determinant of precautionary behavior.

C. *Effects on social relationships*

The fact that SARS is believed by many to be spread through social contact with a person having the disease raises questions about the effects of SARS on social relationships. And, indeed, there have been concerns raised about SARS as a source of discrimination against ethnic groups associated in people's minds with SARS as well as against healthcare workers who have been at high risk of contracting SARS. Newspapers have reported cases in which individuals perceived to possibly be from SARS affected regions or who are Chinese are discriminated against, and there have been reports of healthcare workers being shunned because people were apparently concerned that they might be SARS infected because of their work in healthcare settings. This raises concerns about the effects of SARS on the social fabric. To examine this question, we asked people to indicate their beliefs about how susceptible specific groups of people were to SARS and also how likely they would be to avoid certain people. Respondents coming from both affected and unaffected areas saw the greatest likelihood of having SARS to be for individuals from affected areas. For respondents from unaffected areas, coming from an infected area seemed to be the primary cue that they used to determine if someone might have SARS. For those in affected areas, other cues such as being a healthcare worker, having a fever or coughing were also used. These cues, however, were apparently used less frequently than simply being from a SARS affected area.

Perception of likelihood of a particular type of person having SARS was also closely related to likelihood of avoiding that person, regardless of whether the respondent was from an affected or an unaffected area. Also worry about SARS was associated with both the perception that particular people might have SARS as well as the likelihood of avoiding those people. The more worried someone was about SARS, the greater likelihood they saw for various people to have the disease and the more likely they were to avoid them.

While such reactions are understandable, they also raise concerns about how a condition such as SARS impacts our relationships with others. Social relationships are extremely important to our psychological well being and people particularly need companionship in times of stress. However, avoidance of others on the basis of being perceived to be from a SARS affected area or a healthcare worker deprives those individuals of social contact just when they may need it the most.

For respondents from unaffected areas, coming from an infected area seemed to be the primary cue that they used to determine if someone might have SARS.

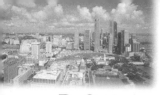

D. Coping

Finally, it is interesting to look at how people coped with the SARS threat. When faced with difficulties, people often utilize a variety to techniques to try to come to grips with the situation and help them cope with it. Research on stress and coping has identified a number of these strategies that people use, which can be roughly classified as problem- or emotion-focused. Problem-focused strategies are concerned with changing the objective situation, whereas emotion-focused techniques aim towards helping the person to adjust to the situation emotionally even if nothing can be done to change the situation itself. A situation like SARS presents a real challenge for people since there is relatively little that most people can do to change the situation other than take recommended precautions. The uncertainty associated with SARS makes things particularly difficult in that it has often been unclear exactly what actions might be effective in warding off SARS. As such people are often forced to use emotion-focused strategies.

To get an idea of how people were coping with their concerns about SARS, we asked our survey respondents about 10 different strategies they might take to deal with the concerns about SARS. Given the limited options that people have for directly influencing the epidemic itself, we expected that emotion-focused strategies would be particularly common and, in fact, three of the four most prevalent strategies reported by survey respondents were concerned with emotion-focused coping. These included wishing that SARS would go away and be done with, trying to keep their feelings about SARS from interfering with other things and trying to see things in a better light. Other strategies used included avoidance, in which the person refused to think about SARS too much, social support where the person talked to someone else about their concerns and planning strategies. For the latter, the person attempted to come up with plans that would lead to the best possible outcome. As such it appeared that people were using appropriate coping strategies for dealing with their SARS concerns. As might be expected, use of these coping strategies was often related to the worries that the person had. For people living in SARS affected areas, there were strong positive relationships between the amount of worry they had about SARS and their use of strategies such as trying to keep their feelings about SARS from interfering with other things, wishing SARS would go away, talking with others about their feelings concerning SARS, and the use of planning strategies.

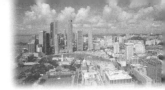

III. Conclusions

The SARS outbreak presented the general public with a number of challenges and highlights the psychological responses that people have to illness. A major factor in people's responses to SARS relates to the high level of uncertainty surrounding the disease. Responding to a deadly disease when there is a great deal of uncertainty about what causes the disease, how it is spread, and the ways one can keep from getting it is bound to create a great deal of anxiety. Fortunately, the probable cause of SARS was identified fairly quickly and relatively straightforward measures to prevent the spread of SARS were implemented speedily. This played a major role in stopping the spread of the disease and also calming people's fears.

Even so, it is very clear that SARS is a source of worry for people, particularly those in affected areas. As we found in our survey that worry is closely related to beliefs that people have about SARS. When people believed that SARS was particularly likely to be spread through various means, such as being near someone with the disease or through poor sanitation or poor personal hygiene, this added to their fears. Also, worry appeared to be fueled by beliefs that particular people were at high risk of getting SARS and also by seeing SARS as being a major problem in various countries, particularly one's own. Fortunately, though, it appears that people were able to keep things in perspective and appeared to be quite accurate in their perception of the threat of SARS relative to other problems they might encounter. Our survey data were reassuring in showing that concerns about SARS seemed to be fairly realistic and not over exaggerated.

In fact, the worries about SARS seemed to be performing a positive function in that they appeared to be motivating people to take appropriate precautions. People who were more worried about SARS were, in fact, the ones who took the most precautions and the most likely to engage in various means to detect possible SARS. It is also reassuring that people, particularly those in affected areas, were taking appropriate precautions. The vast majority of our respondents in affected areas indicated that they were avoiding travel to SARS infected areas, washing their hands more often, taking more care about cleanliness and taking their temperature. It is interesting to note that worry about SARS was not associated with the likelihood of those in affected areas taking actions to determine of they had SARS, but this is most likely due to the strong norms that were established for taking such actions, thus overriding the effects of individual concerns.

It also appears that people coped fairly well with their concerns about SARS although concerns were raised about the effects of SARS on social relationships. Given the high level of uncertainty about SARS and the fact that there was not much that individual laypeople could do about the outbreak, the fact that emotion-focused coping strategies were the most commonly used is appropriate. Emotion-focused approaches tend to be the most effective strategies when there is little that can be objectively done about the situation, since they focus on helping people to look at the situation in more positive ways. Also, it is to be expected that the extent to which people used various coping strategies was related to their concerns about SARS, with those being more concerned also making more use of various coping strategies.

Responses to SARS, however, do raise questions about the effects on social relationships. While, it is understandable that perception that someone might be at risk of being infected with SARS would lead to avoiding that person, a situation such as the SARS outbreak can put considerable strain on the social fabric. For this reason, efforts were made in Singapore and elsewhere to encourage more compassionate and less fearful reactions to SARS patients and their family members and also to show appreciation to healthcare workers, particularly those working directly with SARS patients. These efforts appear to have been successful and in providing social support for those affected by SARS and in motivating people to express their appreciation to healthcare workers.

As of this writing the immediate threat of SARS has passed. Now the challenge relates to consolidating the lessons learned from the SARS outbreak

Emotion-focused approaches tend to be the most effective strategies when there is little that can be objectively done about the situation, since they focus on helping people to look at the situation in more positive ways.

and also keeping people motivated to stay vigilant. With the immediate threat past, worries about SARS are subsiding and since these worries appear to be a major motivator behind preventive measures, it is important to remind people of the possibilities for recurrence so as to encourage them to keep up their guard.

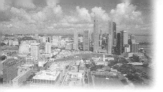

GEORGE D. BISHOP

Dr. George D. Bishop received his Ph.D. in psychology from Yale University and is Professor in the Department of Social Work and Psychology, National University of Singapore. He teaches courses on the psychology of physical health as well as research methods and does research on psychological aspects of health. His work on lay concepts of physical illness as well as psychological and social factors in HIV/AIDS and coronary heart disease has resulted in numerous articles in scholarly journals and book chapters. He is also author of the textbook, *Health Psychology: Integrating Mind and Body*. His current research interests focus on the role of psychosocial factors in CHD as well as lay concepts of physical illness. Prior to coming to NUS in 1991, he taught at the American University in Cairo and the University of Texas at San Antonio.

Correspondence to: Prof. George D. Bishop, E-mail: George_Bishop@nus.edu.sg.

13

Cracking the Genome of the SARS Virus

by Lawrence W. Stanton

In less than a month the complete genetic make up was determined for a previously unidentified life form, a life form that was killing people. The genetic code of the virus that causes SARS had been cracked. The genetic information about this new virus is already providing benefit in the battle to stop and prevent future outbreaks of this public health threat by providing rational approaches to the development of vaccines, therapeutics, and diagnostic tests. This chapter will describe how at the Genome of Institute of Singapore (GIS) the complete genome sequence of the SARS virus was determined, what was learned from the sequence, and how this genetic information is being used to track the spread of SARS. This chapter is not meant to be a scientific review of all that has been published in the scientific community about the sequencing of the SARS genome, but instead provides a first hand account of a human endeavor. For this scientific work was indeed an act of humanity, done by people who lived and worked in Singapore, people who were concerned about the health and well-being of their family and friends as the SARS outbreak

> **Dr. Liu challenged his staff to think creatively about approaches to fight this public health crisis utilizing the considerable technical and intellectual capabilities that resided within the institute.**

unfolded. Scientists often work on rather obscure bits of nature, sometimes offering little practical benefit. With SARS, the research was different — it felt personal and it felt urgent.

The Challenge to Sequence the SARS Virus

On Monday morning of March 31, 2003 the scientists were arriving for work at the Genome Institute of Singapore (GIS). They expected to resume their ongoing experiments on stem cells, cancer, human genetics, or comparative genomics, but this quickly changed. That morning the Executive Director of GIS, Dr. Edison Liu, assembled his team leaders to announce a new directive — a commitment to do research on SARS. Dr. Liu challenged his staff to think creatively about approaches to fight this public health crisis utilizing the considerable technical and intellectual capabilities that resided within the institute. By the end of the week, 50 scientists at GIS, approximately half of the scientific staff, were working on some aspect of the SARS problem. There was a major commitment of resources to sequence the virus genome, develop diagnostic tests, and characterize the virus for development of therapies and vaccines. The other projects would continue, but with lower priority than the SARS work. Though a good portion of our work involved vaccines and therapeutics, the focus here will be on the work directed towards sequencing the genome of the SARS virus and the subsequent analysis of genetic diversity among different strains of the SARS virus.

The heart of any genome institute is its DNA sequencing operation. At GIS the sequencing operation occupies one-fourth of the lab space and employees nearly one-fourth of the research staff. The sequencing operation is a combination of quiet, creative, and hand-crafted molecular biology at one end, and high capacity production line work at the other. As one enters the sequencing labs the production operation is clearly evident. There are robots picking, placing, and transferring reagents step by step in automated and high throughput fashion. Some of these robotic devices are large and noisy, and the lab can feel like a factory when all this equipment is running at full speed. Then there are the rather inconspicuous automated DNA sequencing machines, six of them clustered together in the lab. A small flashing light is the only indication that the machine is running. Very quietly these machines precisely determine the sequence of the bits of DNA that have been loaded into the device by the scientist.

The sequencing operation is led by Dr. Ruan Yijun and Dr. Wei Chia Lin, who have assembled a team that can adroitly handle the molecular biology, the production aspects of the sequencing operation, and the computational analysis. When Dr. Liu decided to devote resources to getting the sequencing done, it was with the knowledge that this team was fully capable of bringing success to such a project. The sequencing engines were ready to roll — they just needed DNA molecules to sequence. The challenge was to devise strategies that would put these sequencing engines to work.

The first challenge was to find a good source of the SARS virus. The rate of achieving success was dependent upon the amount and purity of the virus. The virus would be provided by Dr. Ling Ai Ee and her research team from the Department of Pathology at the Singapore General Hospital. Dr. Ling had been seeking to identify the agent that causes SARS. She and her colleagues were among the first groups to recognize viral particles in the infected lung tissue of patients who had died from SARS. Highly magnified images of the virus taken by electron microscopy revealed a distinctive structural feature. The virus appeared as a round particle with spike-like projections reminiscent of a crown. This was a substantial clue to the type of virus that causes SARS. The size and shape of the virus was suggestive that it was a coronavirus, so named for its distinctive crown shape. Knowledge that the suspect cause of SARS was a coronavirus was helpful in the development

The sequencing operation is led by Dr. Ruan Yijun and Dr. Wei Chia Lin.

> **The first challenge was to find a good source of the SARS virus. The virus would be provided by Dr. Ling Ai Ee and her research team from the Department of Pathology at the Singapore General Hospital.**

of diagnostic tests. However, to complete the sequence of the virus a rich source was still required and the source would be from cultured monkey cells. It turned out that the SARS virus did not infect any of the standard human cell types that are often utilized to propagate human viruses in the lab. Dr. Ling's group continued to test numerous cell types, which included a cell line that originated from an African green monkey, known as the Vero cells. When respiratory samples collected from SARS patients were added to the Vero cells, the cells showed signs of infection. Microscopic examination of the cultured cells confirmed they were infected and producing coronaviruses indistinguishable from those seen in SARS patient samples. This breakthrough provided the means to produce large quantities of virus and material that was suitable for sequencing.

Devising a Strategy to Sequence the SARS Virus Genome

There were a number of strategies available to sequence the SARS genetic material that had been isolated from the Vero cells. Because the exact genomic sequence was not known, direct molecular approaches such as PCR amplification could not be used. The key, therefore, was to mine the viral material for exact genetic sequence that could be used as "anchors" for large scale sequencing. The sequencing group attacked the sequencing from several directions. One strategy that proved successful was the "shot-gun" approach. This approach has been successfully applied to sequence several complete genomes, including those of the mouse and human, which are 100,000 times larger than the SARS viral genome. With shot-gun sequencing, the genome is first chopped up into many short fragments. Then the entire genome sequence is ascertained by sequencing each of the smaller fragments. Next, the individual bits of DNA sequence are assembled to reveal the entire genome sequence. The assembly process will succeed only if sufficient bits of sequence are available that produce a full complement of overlapping sequences. It is the overlaps of common sequences from individual fragments that permit the correct assembly of all the pieces. In practice, 5-fold more sequence is determined in 500 nucleotide fragments to generate a fully assembled genome sequence. Thus, for a 30,000 nucleotide genome, the size of the SARS virus, a manageable number of 300 individual fragments would be sequenced and assembled. However, there were some complications in determining the SARS genome sequence.

As Dr. Ruan and his team began applying the shot-gun strategy, some questions remained unanswered. The team was confident in the approach, for it had been successful with many large genome sequencing projects. However, the size of the SARS viral genome was not known. It was expected to be similar in size to other coronaviruses, approximately 30,000 nucleotides. However, the SARS virus genome could be larger, which would require more fragments to be sequenced and assembled. The second and bigger issue was that isolated samples of virus would be contaminated with RNA from the Vero cells, the host cells that produce the virus. The amount of contamination was not known, but any contaminants would increase the number of fragments that must be sequenced. If there was only 10% contamination, that would be no problem, as only 10% more fragments would be required. However, it was distinctly possible that there was 10–100 times more Vero cell-associated RNA than that from the virus, which would seriously amplify the number of fragments that must be sequenced. So as the team began the shot-gun strategy, they figured minimally 300 fragments must be sequenced, but possibly it would take 3000–30,000 individual sequences to be determined.

Another complicating issue was that SARS was likely a coronavirus, and coronaviral genomes are made of RNA. Most genomes are DNA-based, which is compatible with high throughput sequencing operations. RNA genomes have been sequenced, but an extra step is needed to convert the RNA into DNA. The extra step, called reverse transcription, can be somewhat tricky. The concern was that certain regions of the viral RNA would not efficiently convert to DNA, which would leave large holes in the sequence and compromise the assembly process. In addition, unlike DNA, RNA is notoriously unstable. A sample of RNA can be quickly degraded by nuclease

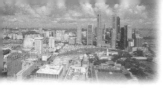

proteins that are present everywhere, including on researchers' finger tips. RNA samples that are degraded will not yield sequence data and so great care must be taken during preparation of viral RNA. None of the complicating issues were likely to be insurmountable, but they could slow the progress — perhaps a little or perhaps a lot. The team knew the biggest issue was the uncertainty about the quantity and quality of the starting RNA material. To mitigate the uncertainty, several independently isolated samples were processed simultaneously. This added to the workload, but was necessary to reduce the risk of working with a single sample of unknown condition.

SARS Virus Samples are Obtained

On April 4, 2003 the team received its first RNA samples from Dr. Ling Ai Ee's group. Some of the samples were taken from two patients who had died of SARS. It is not possible to ignore the fact that these samples came from a Singaporean who succumbed to an infectious disease that was not under control. It is difficult to remain unemotional as one uses these samples to ostensibly identify the cause of death. Everyone at GIS had been reading the newspapers daily, hearing details about the latest victim who succumbed to the virus. The samples received in the lab are given a coded identification number and all details of the individual remain unknown to the team to protect the privacy of the patients and their families. Nonetheless, we wondered, was this sample taken from the male doctor we read about who contracted the disease from his patient, or perhaps from the elderly woman who died after exposure through a chance contact with a SARS infected person? We wondered who these people were and knew that the loved ones were mourning their loss. It reminded us that this virus could kill and that we were all potential victims of its indiscriminate infections.

There was also concern about the safety of handling the samples. Very little was known about the SARS virus at the time. Clearly, it was infectious and could be spread, but the mode of transmission and the ease of spread was still unclear. Dr. Ling's group performed all their work under stringent containment measures, which they routinely utilize in their work to identify infectious agents at the Virology Section of the Singapore General Hospital. The Singapore Ministry of Health correctly insisted that SARS infectious

Biosafety level 3 (BSL3) is required for laboratories that handle pathogens, such as SARS virus, that spread by aerosol routes. A BSL3 lab must be equipped with secondary containment devices that prevent escape of the pathogen into the environment.

material would be handled under containment conditions known as BSL3. The heightened level of containment was absolutely necessary to protect the researchers and to ensure that no additional spread of the SARS epidemic would occur as a result of inadequate laboratory safety measures at a time when containment of the outbreak was the highest priority.

Biosafety level 3 (BSL3) is required for laboratories that handle pathogens, such as SARS virus, that spread by aerosol routes. A BSL3 lab must be equipped with secondary containment devices that prevent escape of the pathogen into the environment. Thus, all personnel must wear personal protective devices such as disposable gowns, gloves, and face shields. Most of the work is done in fully exhausted Biosafety cabinets that provide containment of airborne infectious material. All waste materials from a BSL3 lab are autoclaved (heated under pressure) before removal from the lab to destroy residual pathogens. In addition, the room is maintained under negative air pressure in conjunction with high efficiency particle (HEPA) filtration to prevent airborne dissemination of pathogens.

A BSL3 facility was available at the Virology Section of the Singapore General Hospital for handling SARS infected samples. Dr. Ling's staff were fully trained to handle such infectious material within the BSL3 lab. Research on SARS would not be possible without the expertise and dedication of staff like those in Dr. Ling's team who put themselves at risk so that we may understand this virus and better control the epidemic. In order to sequence the SARS virus genome, sufficient amounts of viral RNA had to be extracted from infectious material, and this task was handled with aplomb by Dr. Ling's team, in particular, Se Thoe Su Yun, Chan Kwai Peng, and Lynette Oon Lin Ean. This team prepared the RNA from the patient samples and transferred the RNA to GIS to initiate the genome sequencing.

Another ongoing research effort, being led by Dr. Ren Ee Chee at GIS, was to establish a diagnostic test for SARS.

From the initial set of samples, it was evident that there were greater amounts of viral RNA in the samples that had been propagated on Vero tissue culture cells. The viral RNA isolated directly from the lung tissues was of insufficient quantity to generate high quality sequence. However, preliminary analysis indicated that the RNA from SARS infected Vero cells contained sufficient amounts of viral RNA. These assessments were possible because of some additional work ongoing at GIS to identify the SARS virus.

Another ongoing research effort, being led by Dr. Ren Ee Chee at GIS, was to establish a diagnostic test for SARS. Within the SARS Diagnostics team was Dr. Lisa Ng, a bright and energetic post-doctoral fellow, who coincidently had worked on coronaviruses as part of her doctoral training. Dr. Ng and Dr. Ren had correctly predicted a region of the SARS viral genome that would be most similar to known coronaviruses. They were able to develop key reagents that were utilized in a method called PCR, for polymerase chain reaction, to amplify a particular region of the SARS virus genome, which at the time was still completely unknown. The so-called primers they designed amplified by PCR a short stretch of DNA from the SARS infected lung samples. The short stretch was sequenced and gave GIS their first peek at the SARS virus genome. Although the sequence was relatively small, only 450 nucleotides of the entire 30,000 nucleotide genome, it was sufficient to identify a new member of the coronavirus family, which underscored the need to complete the sequence of the entire genome. The ability to detect SARS virus RNA with this newly developed PCR method was very helpful for the sequencing project. We could now test samples to determine if the SARS virus was present and how much RNA was in the sample. Many patient samples were tested, including blood, respiratory exudates, and stool, as well as lung tissue taken from individuals who died from SARS. It was clear that the highest concentration of virus was in the Vero cell cultures and efforts were focused upon this source of material for sequencing.

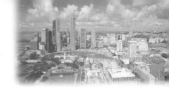

Sequencing the SARS Virus Genome

The most delicate part of any sequencing project is to construct high quality libraries of DNA templates from the viral RNA samples. Dr. Wei Chia Lin is an expert in this field and it was her mission to construct these libraries to make the sequencing possible. The SARS viral genome is a single strand of RNA, which had to be converted to double-stranded DNA for sequencing. Conversion of RNA to DNA is a standard trick of the trade in molecular biology. The process is known as reverse transcription because it is the opposite of transcription, a fundamental process of living cells whereby a copy of RNA is generated from DNA. Transcription and reverse transcription convert the chemical composition of the nucleic acid, deoxyribose versus ribose, without changing the sequence of the nucleotides during the conversion. Therefore, the sequence of double-stranded DNA that has been reverse transcribed from SARS viral RNA will be identical. Although RNA molecules can be sequenced directly, the methodology is more cumbersome than DNA sequencing. The conversion of SARS viral RNA to DNA was accomplished by reverse transcriptase, an enzymatic protein that can be purchased from specialty vendors of molecular biology reagents. Reverse transcriptase requires a DNA primer, which dictates where the enzyme is to begin reading the RNA strand and producing the DNA copy of that RNA.

For the sequencing project it was important to have all the viral RNA converted to DNA, but not necessarily in one continuous piece. So a mixture of DNA primers was used that permitted random priming of the reverse transcriptase along the viral RNA genome. The end result was a mixture of

The most delicate part of any sequencing project is to construct high quality libraries of DNA templates from the viral RNA samples. Dr. Wei Chia Lin is an expert in this field and it was her mission to construct these libraries to make the sequencing possible.

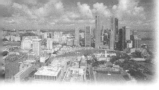

DNA molecules that collectively covered the entire genome of the SARS virus. To facilitate the next steps in the sequencing process, the exceedingly small amount of DNA fragments were amplified using PCR. The next step was to produce a library of bacteria that contains the entire SARS viral genome in fragments. In the library there are millions of bacteria, each containing a single DNA fragment that originated from the mixture of fragments generated in the previous steps. The utility of the bacterial library is that a single bacterium can be grown into a large isolated colony, which thereby expands the amount of each viral DNA fragment to generate enough material for the sequencing process.

With the construction of the SARS virus library, it was now time to determine the sequence of the individual fragments, which would then be assembled to generate a complete genome sequence. Mr. Herve Thoreau and Mr. Landri Lim managed all aspects of the sequencing production operation: prepared DNA samples from bacteria, performed sequencing reactions, ran DNA sequencing instruments, collected raw sequence data, and assembled the complete sequences. Mr. Thoreau, Mr. Lim, and the production team had been anxiously awaiting samples to run through the bank of DNA sequencers. DNA was prepared from 2000 bacterial colonies isolated from the SARS virus library and then sequenced. This is a modest number of fragments to sequence for the operation at GIS. The samples were loaded onto the machine and the team nervously awaited the results. The initial results would inform the team about the quality of their libraries. They would have a good idea if the genome sequence would be obtained quickly or would require substantially more effort and time. After two hours, the prepared samples were sequenced and the raw data were streaming off the sequencing machines. The data were automatically routed to a computer where the sequence was compiled and analyzed by computer scientist, Jer-Min Chia and group leader A/P Prasanna Kolatkar. It seemed as though all of GIS was collectively holding their breath.

The initial results were in and they were quite encouraging. It was assessed that approximately one half of the fragments sequenced had not been derived from Vero cells. Many of these fragments shared sequence similarity with other known coronaviruses. This meant that much of the library was likely derived from the SARS virus and suggested that the complete sequence could be assembled from the library of fragments that were in hand. It was estimated that 5,000 individual colonies would need to be sequenced to complete the

The team did finish the sequence of a Singapore SARS virus that week and on April 19, 2003 that sequence, along with four other completed SARS genomes, was posted on the GIS web site and submitted to GenBank, a public sequence database.

task. This was a manageable number and could be completed in about two days with the sequencing operation running at top speed. Another day or two would likely be needed to polish a few trouble spots in the sequence. The team wasted no time in proceeding; in fact, it had already been moving forward in anticipation of positive results from the preliminary experiments. The team was tired, but the positive data generated enthusiasm that provided a boost of energy to the sleep-deprived group. In a few more days they figured to have the sequence completed.

The First Complete Genome Sequence of the SARS Virus

On April 12, 2003, as the GIS sequencing team was pushing to the finish line there was news that a team from the British Columbia Genome Science Center in Canada had completed the genome sequence of the SARS virus. We knew there were other groups working to complete the SARS viral genome. GIS had hoped to be the first to complete the sequencing of the killer virus. The team was disappointed that in spite of their heroic efforts they would not be the first. Then the next day, a team from the Center for Disease Control in the United States announced that they, too, had a complete sequence of the SARS coronavirus, so GIS would not even be second to complete the SARS viral sequence, which brought more disappointment to the GIS team. This was, after all, how science is conducted, one of progressively answering important questions. Though someone came first with the sequence, there were equally critical questions that now needed to be answered. The strategy, therefore, was immediately redirected to attack the next most important question, that of genetic mutations in the virus. In order to devise the best diagnostics and therapeutics, this information was critical. The team did finish the sequence of a Singapore SARS virus that week and on April 19, 2003 that sequence, along with four other completed SARS genomes (described below), was posted on the GIS web site and submitted to GenBank, a public sequence database. It was a tremendous accomplishment for a fledgling genome institute and the team was proud of their work. In just two weeks from the time the virus samples were in hand, GIS had determined the complete sequence of a novel virus, one that was killing people and spreading fear in communities throughout the world. Their work would help improve the chances of establishing solid clinical detection of the virus in patient sample and lead to advances in developing vaccines and therapeutics to stop SARS.

There was much excitement about the newly revealed sequence of the SARS virus. Scientists at GIS and elsewhere now had a good look at this virus at its most fundamental level, its complete genetic code. There were many questions that we had about this virus and now the sequence was available to provide some answers. A couple of conclusions were quickly drawn from the complete genome sequence of the SARS virus. The SARS virus genome has the typical features of a coronavirus, but is clearly unique compared with all previously identified coronaviruses. All other coronaviruses have been grouped into three families based on sequence similarity. The sequence of the SARS virus does not appear to fit preferentially into any one of the existing families and has been proposed to be the founder of a fourth family. There was anticipation that the sequence of the SARS virus would provide clues to the origin of this virus. If the SARS virus was more similar to coronaviruses known to infect birds, then this strain may have originated and perhaps remains within a species of bird. However, the sequence gave no strong support for any particular species of origin and it remains an open question as to where the virus came from.

The SARS viral genome, like other coronaviruses, contains genes that encode for proteins necessary for the virus to infect its host and replicate (Fig. 1). These include replicases 1(a) and 1(b), which are essential for viral replication. Proteins that form the outer surface of the virus and mediate the entry of virus into cells are encoded by the spike (S), envelope (E), membrane (M), and nucleocapsid (N) genes. Several other genes are predicted based on the presence of open reading frames that likely encode for proteins, but the function of these proteins remains unknown.

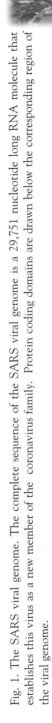
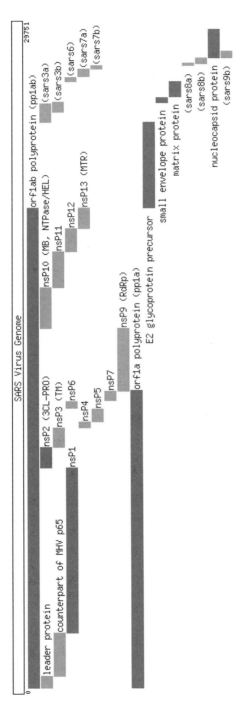

Fig. 1. The SARS viral genome. The complete sequence of the SARS viral genome is a 29,751 nucleotide long RNA molecule that establishes this virus as a new member of the coronavirus family. Protein coding domains are drawn below the corresponding region of the viral genome.

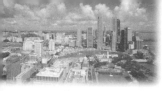

Sequence Diversity among Strains of the SARS Virus

The team at GIS was disappointed that they were not the first to publish the genome sequence of the SARS virus, but it was not time to dwell on this setback. It was time to push hard on phase 2. The second phase for sequencing of the SARS virus was already planned while the first sequence was being determined. The plan was to determine several distinct SARS viral sequences and compare the sequences with one another. This was important to learn about the genetic diversity of the virus. Was there more than one strain of SARS virus? Was there a unique genetic feature of viruses that killed the patient? Did the so-called super-spreaders of the SARS develop and disperse a mutant version of SARS coronavirus that was more contagious? Did the SARS virus mutate quickly as it spread in the population, which could lead to subsequent outbreaks as occurs with influenza? To get answers to these questions, we needed more sequences of the SARS viruses.

In phase 2, the GIS team would complete the sequence of five individual isolates of the SARS virus. While the first sequence was being generated at GIS, Dr. Ling and her colleagues had provided four additional SARS viral isolates. Among the five viral isolates was the first Singapore resident with SARS (index case), who contracted the disease in Hong Kong at the Hotel Metropole. Three of the viral isolates, second generation Singapore cases, came from patients who contracted SARS directly from the index case. Virus from a third generation Singapore SARS case, who contracted the disease from a second generation case, was also available for sequencing. All five viral genomes would be completely sequenced using a new strategy.

Once the first SARS virus sequence was available, it was no longer necessary to perform shot-gun sequencing. A more streamlined strategy was now possible. The new strategy was to specifically amplify the entire genome in 30 fragments of approximately 1000 bases each. Each of the fragments could then be sequenced quickly and assembled into the complete genome sequence. With this strategy, a new SARS viral isolate could be completely sequenced in less than a week. In fact, several complete genomes could be done simultaneously in the same amount of time. Within a week of the first reported sequence of a SARS virus, GIS had amassed five new complete genome sequences.

The sequences of all five SARS strains collected from patients in Singapore were compared. The pressing question was whether this virus had mutated

Indeed there was clear evidence of mutation when the five strains of SARS virus from Singapore were compared.

rapidly as it passed from one individual to the next. A high mutation rate could be problematic from a public health perspective. If the SARS virus mutated quickly, it might become more virulent, though it might also evolve to a less virulent form. In addition, if the virus alters quickly, SARS could reemerge in people who had already developed antibodies against SARS, which would create recurring cycle of outbreaks in the world population. Viruses that mutate rapidly such as HIV, which causes AIDS, have been notoriously resistant to vaccine development. For these reasons, it was important to understand the SARS virus at the genetic level and to gauge its rate of change through the epidemic. The sequence of the five Singapore isolates would be very helpful as they came from three successive generations of SARS transmission where the contact history was well established.

Indeed, there was clear evidence of mutation when the five strains of SARS virus from Singapore were compared. The three primary contacts had 5, 3, and 3 genetic differences from the index case (7 single point changes and 4 small deletions). This works out to be a mutation rate of approximately 0.01% per generation. There were four differences between the index case and the third generation contact. (The direct contact of this third generation case was not available for study.) These data indicate that there is not a high rate of mutation or a propensity for major genetic rearrangements within the RNA genome of the SARS virus. The genomes of RNA viruses, such as HIV, have high rates of mutation because the machinery that replicates RNA is less reliable than that utilized to replicate DNA. Nonetheless, these data indicate that the SARS virus does mutate and this study reinforces the need to monitor genetic diversity of the virus as it spreads through the population.

Sequences of other SARS viral genomes were being elucidated in labs around the world. The sequences of other strains from outside of Singapore would give a broader picture of the genetic diversity of the SARS virus. By early June of 2003, there were 18 complete or nearly complete sequences available in public databases. We were interested to compare all of these

235

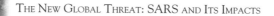

> ## We were interested to compare all of these sequences, which was a computational challenge. That challenge was met by Dr. Philip Long, Head of the Computational Biology Group at GIS.

sequences, which was a computational challenge. That challenge was met by Dr. Philip Long, Head of the Computational Biology Group at GIS, and a talented graduate student in the group, Vega Vinsensius. The CompBio group had been engaged in the SARS sequencing project from the start. They had compared all the known coronaviruses for areas of sequence conservation that aided the GIS team to quickly isolate and sequence a 3000 nucleotide region of the SARS virus several weeks before the complete SARS genome had been cracked. Now they had genome sequences for 18 SARS virus strains and they were eager to compare them. They discovered 150 variant positions (138 single position changes and 12 small deletions) among all the sequences, which amounts to a mutation rate of approximately 0.03%. The number of differences across all strains was about 3-fold higher than the rate of variation observed among the five Singapore strains. The greater variation among all strains relative to the Singapore strains is to be expected since the Singapore strains were among three generations, while the number of generations of virus worldwide is much broader, though undetermined. It remains unclear what impact these mutations have on the virus, though many of the changes would affect the structure of certain viral proteins. It should be noted that some of these apparent differences were likely the result of errors in sequencing. Other variants may arise during culturing of the virus in Vero cells and were not present in the virus taken from SARS patients.

The Computational Biology group at GIS noticed that there are certain variants that occur more than once among the 18 isolates. Some of these common variant sequences are interesting in that they segregate with geographical routes of transmission. Most notable are five positions in the sequence, bases 9404, 17564, 21721, 22222, and 27827. These five loci are either of the sequence TTGTT or CGACC in 17 of the 18 strains (Fig. 2). There are 12 strains with the TTGTT genotype and five strains with the

CGACC genotype. The TTGTT sequence is present in all the strains that can be linked to the Hotel Metropole in Hong Kong, a site that is well documented to have been a focal point for the spread of SARS to several countries. The distinctive TTGTT signature is present in all the five Singapore strains, plus one each from Hong Kong, Canada, and Vietnam (all the patients in these cases had contracted SARS in the Hotel Metropole). The strains that had the CGACC genotype had no connection with the hotel in Hong Kong. Thus, the sequence at these five positions represent signatures (named here the "Guangdong" and "Hong Kong" signatures) of the virus that can be traced to that particular regional outbreak.

Other common sequence signatures emerged from the data that also correlate with presumed routes of viral transmission. For instance, in the four strains collected at similar times in Beijing, the sequence is TGT at positions 9854, 19838, and 27243. In most other strains collected outside of Beijing, the sequence is CAC. The TGT genotype at these sites represents a signature ("Beijing" signature) for the Beijing cluster and distinguishes the virus from strains isolated in other parts of China and Asia (Fig. 2). One strain of SARS, ZJ01, which was isolated in China, has the "Hong Kong" signature and another strain, HKU-HW1, which was isolated in Hong Kong, has the "Guangdong" signature. The signature sequences indicate that transmission of SARS to these individuals likely occurred from a non-local contact. It would be of interest to determine if these cases involved travel outside their local region or recent contact with a traveler that might explain the source of the strain they carry.

Analysis of the Singapore sequences elucidated another signature sequence ("Singapore" signature). Among four of the five Singapore strains, there was a T at position 19084 (Fig. 2). Outside of Singapore, this position was typically C. Thus, this signature reflects a strain of virus that was spread by one of the index cases (SIN2500) in Singapore. Surprisingly, the third generation Singapore case (SIN2679) lacks the T at this position. One possible explanation is that in the transmission of the virus to this individual, there was a mutation that reversed the sequence that defines the "Singapore" signature. However, another possible scenario is that the route of transmission to SIN2679 was from a different index case. Sequence data of the other individuals within this group of contacts is required to elaborate on this issue. Also of note is that the "Singapore" signature is present in a strain isolated

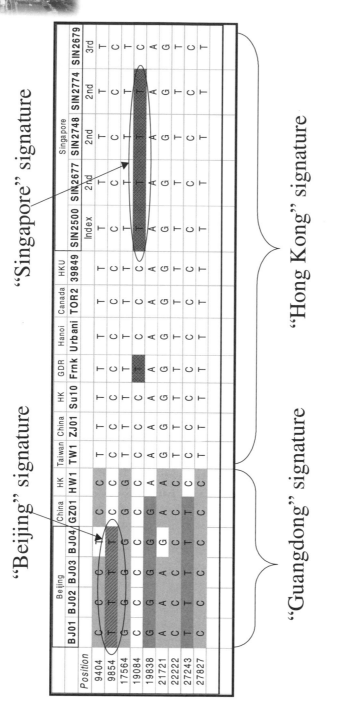

Fig. 2. Genetic signatures of the SARS virus. Sequence variations that occur in at least 4 SARS strains are indicated. Shaded boxes show the variant nucleotide at the indicated position on the SARS genome (numbered according to TOR2 sequence). The names and case locations are given for each of the 18 strains. Common sequence variants among the strains, which segregate to geographic regions, define genetic signatures that can be used to distinguish individual isolates of SARS virus.

from a patient in Frankfurt, Germany. In this instance, the signature sequence provides confirmation of the presumed transmission history as the Frankfurt individual had had contact with a Singaporean SARS patient. The one sequence from a Taiwan isolate of the SARS virus displays the "Hong Kong" signature (Fig. 2). It will be interesting to determine with additional sequences if the large outbreak in Taiwan was derived exclusively from the "Hong Kong" strain or if there are also cases with the "Guangdong" strain.

Genetic signatures of the SARS virus will be of use in tracing routes of transmission and will be helpful in tracing contact histories, which has been extremely useful in containing the spread of SARS. For example, if a resident of Singapore who recently traveled to Hong Kong develops SARS, it would be important to know where the virus was contracted. Then health authorities could concentrate contact tracing in the appropriate locations. This could also reduce the number of people who would be placed in quarantine. These genetic signatures would also be useful in confirming the route of transmission. For instance, it would be important to confirm that a presumed spread of SARS from patient to healthcare worker did indeed occur. Establishing a common genetic signature between the presumed spreader and recipient would substantially decrease the likelihood that transmission occurred in the community or elsewhere in the hospital. In addition, the knowledge of the sequence variations allowed Dr. Ren Ee Chee, Martin Hibberd, and Lisa Ng to develop the most robust nucleic acid based diagnostic test, one that would not be affected by genetic mutations. This information has also been used to direct vaccine development.

Conclusion

The battle against SARS has been waged on many fronts. The worldwide campaign to contain the disease has brought together clinicians, epidemiologists, researchers, and government officials in the fight against a common opponent. The initial success to curtail the spread of SARS was made possible by groups and individuals working together. We saw unusual degrees of cooperation across political, social, and professional boundaries. In an incredibly short period of time the virus that causes SARS was identified, isolated, and its genetic code revealed. The ability to sequence the complete genome of a novel organism in a few short weeks is testament to the advances made in molecular biology over the past 50 years since Watson and Crick first elucidated the structure of DNA.

The successful sequencing of the SARS viral genome has provided certain short term benefits and many long term benefits shall follow. The viral sequence provides a complete inventory of all the proteins that SARS virus produces in order to survive by infection and replication in its human host. Knowledge of these viral proteins will provide us with the opportunity to stop the spread of SARS. Some of these proteins are already being utilized in the production of vaccines. A few encoded by the virus are excellent targets for development of drugs to treat and save lives of SARS patients. The genome sequence has launched production of diagnostic methods that provide clinical confirmation of a disease whose symptoms are common in non-SARS patients.

The ability to rapidly sequence new isolates of the SARS virus has now provided an unprecedented opportunity to track the spread of viral infection. Molecular signatures within the viral genomes provide the molecular epidemiologist with fingerprints of the culprit that has spread the disease. Routes and modes of SARS transmission can be established and confirmed, which will improve the management of SARS by the effective strategies of isolation and containment of infected individuals and their recent contacts. A continued spirit of cooperation among countries and professions is needed to insure that the most effective measures are applied to contain, or perhaps eliminate, SARS.

Acknowledgements

The spirit of cooperation and dedication was never more apparent than within the Sequencing Group at the Genome Institute of Singapore. A special thank you is extended to these members of the GIS team, and to those who were mentioned in the text, who have contributed to the SARS sequencing effort: Agatha Susila, Bhinu V.S., Emmanuel Lambert, Frans Verhoef, Gayathri Balasundaram, Joanne Leong, Joshy George, Kok Wui Lim, Kuo Ping Chiu, Lim Kuo Foong, Lin Su, Marie Wong, Melvyn Tan, Ng Su Peng, Ooi Poh Ling, Patrick Ng, Sanjay Gupta, Serene Lee, Yeo Ailing, and Zang Tao.

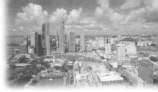

LAWRENCE W. STANTON

Dr. Lawrence W. Stanton is Senior Group Leader and SARS Project Coordinator at the Genome Institute of Singapore. He obtained his Ph.D. from the State University of New York, Stony Brook, USA. His research include human embryonic stem cell differentiation and regulation of gene expression.

Professional history:

2001–2002	Director of Functional Genomics, Geron Corporation, USA
2000–2001	Project Leader DNA microarrays, Agilent Technologies, USA
1990–2000	Group Leader Genomics Technologies, Scios Inc., USA
1985–1989	Post-doctoral Fellow, Lab of J. Michael Bishop, USA

Awards and honors:

1995	NIH Small Business Innovative Research (SBIR) Grant
1989	Research Award, American Assoc. Cancer Research
1987–1989	NIH Senior Fellowship
1985–1987	Leukemia Society of America Fellowship

Publications (selected, of 32 total):

1. L.W. Stanton, G. Endemann *et al.*, *J Biol Chem* **267**: 22446–22451, (1992).
2. G. Endemann, L.W. Stanton *et al.*, *J Biol Chem* **268**: 11811–11816, (1993).
3. T.J. Aitman, L.W. Stanton, *et al.*, *Nature Genetics* **21**: 76–83, (1999).
4. L.W. Stanton, L.J. *et al.*, *Circulation Research* **86**: 939–945, (2000).
5. L.W. Stanton, *Trends in Cardiovascular Medicine* **11**: 49–54 (2001). *Invited Review*.
6. Wallace CA, *et al.*, Stanton LW and Aitman TJ, *Mamm enome* **13**(4): 194–197, (2002).
7. Identification of molecular markers of human embryonic stem cells by gene expression analysis. Stanton LW *et al.*, submitted (2003).
8. Genomic analysis of human embryonic stem cells. Stanton LW, *et al.*, in preparation (2003).

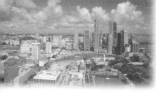

9. Comparative full-length genome sequence analysis of 14 SARS coronavirus isolates and common mutations associated with putative origins of infection. Ruan YJ, et al., *Lancet* 2003.

Contact Information: Genome Institute of Singapore, 1 Science Park Road, The Capricorn #5-01, Singapore 117528, Phone: (65) 6827 5280, Email: gisslw@nus.edu

14

The Infection Control Response to SARS in Hospitals and Institutions

by *Paul Ananth Tambyah*

Introduction

The severe acute respiratory syndrome (SARS) is a newly recognized coronavirus infection that emerged in East Asia with subsequent global spread.[1-3] Hospitals have been the major foci of infection especially in Singapore[4] and Canada[5] where more than three-quarters of cases have occurred in visitors, healthcare workers (HCWs) and other patients in the same rooms of unrecognized SARS patients. In February 2003, reports began emerging on ProMed Mail of an outbreak of atypical pneumonia in Guangdong

---

This chapter represents my own opinions and in no way reflect the views of any members of the National University Hospital or the National University of Singapore.

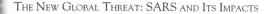

> **One of the first unusual aspects of this emerging infection was the recognition that healthcare workers (HCW) were uniquely susceptible to the then unknown etiologic agent.**

province in China.[6] The World Health Organization had requested for information about this outbreak, but it did not really hit the headlines globally until early March 2003. The global dissemination of SARS is believed to have begun from the Hotel M in Hongkong where a physician from Guandong stayed for one day.[7] At least 16 individuals, none of whom reportedly had direct contact with him, who were living on the ninth floor of the hotel, were subsequently infected with SARS. They traveled onwards to their homes or next destinations in the United States, Canada, Singapore, Hongkong and Ireland sparking off epidemics of varying degrees of severity in each of those countries mainly in hospitals but also in their respective communities.

Nosocomial Spread and the Proliferation of Guidelines

One of the first unusual aspects of this emerging infection was the recognition that healthcare workers (HCW) were uniquely susceptible to the then unknown etiologic agent. As soon as SARS was recognized as a nosocomial infection, guidelines were issued by various authorities including the World Health Organization,[8] the United States Centers for Disease Control and Prevention[9] and the Hongkong Health Authority,[10] Health Canada,[11] Ministries of Health of Singapore,[12] Malaysia,[13] among others. The key features of these guidelines are summarized in Table 1. It is important to recognize that in the beginning, there was no information about what was the agent responsible for this infection or its mode of transmission, hence a tendency to "over-protect". As the epidemic evolved, so did the guidelines and these are constantly updated and might indeed be out of date by the time this is read. All are published on the Internet[8–13] and the reader is encouraged to review the websites for the latest information.

Table 1   Guidelines for Infection Control for SARS in the Hospital Setting

	WHO	US CDC	Health Canada	Hongkong HA	Singapore MOH
Personal Protective Equipment					
Mask	N100 preferred, fit testing ideal	N95 for all suspect	N95 or equivalent	Surgical mask or N95 mask	Fit tested N95 or equivalent
Eye protection	Eye protection for all suspect cases	Eye protection for all contact with SARS pts	For direct patient care, aerosol/splash inducing procedures	Eye shield	Goggles or face shields for patient contact
Gown	With apron for all	Gown for all suspect		Gown	Gown
Glove	Glove for all suspect	Glove for all suspect, standard precautions for all patients		Gloves	Glove
Intubation/high risk respiratory procedures	"Particular attention should be paid"	Airborne isolation room, N95 or greater, consider PAPR	Limit personnel, duration, no additional PPE	Good ventilation, avoid nebulisers, Full PPE for aerosol generating areas	PAPR mandatory
Administrative/Environmental Controls					
Visitors	Full PPE, discouraged	As per airborne isolation	Not allowed	Not allowed	Not allowed
Disinfection	"Broad spectrum disinfectant"	Any EPA registered disinfectant for low/intermediate level cleaning	"Frequent cleaning"	Daily with 1:49 hypochlorite or 70% alcohol,1:5 bleach if heavily soiled	Daily with phenolic or alcohol based product
Airflow/Isolation	Preferably negative pressure room, alternatives include single room and if not available, cohort with independent air supply	Negative pressure for all suspect	Negative pressure preferred, single room alternative	Preferably from low to high risk	Preferably negative pressure, as per WHO
Routine Laboratory Work	Standard precautions, BSL-2	Standard precautions, BSL-2	Full PPE, BSL-2	Class 1 biosafety cabinet	Not specified
Remains	Not specified	Full PPE, standard burial/cremation	Gloves, no special precautions, full PPE for post-mortems	Double bag, category 2*, full PPE including N95 or PAPR	Full PPE, 24 hour cremation unless exceptional circumstance

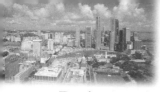

Background: Fears of Pandemic Influenza

It has long been recognized that the world is "overdue" for an influenza pandemic and in fact, in February, there had been a small cluster of cases of the dreaded avian influenza in a Hongkong family who had traveled to mainland China.[14] One of the Singaporean women who returned from the Hotel M was indeed isolated as a possible case of avian influenza in one of Singapore's large general hospitals and no secondary cases resulted from her. Because of the concerns about possible avian influenza or some unknown pathogen with an uncertain mode of transmission, most of the initial strategies devised for the prevention and control of SARS were directed against a highly contagious airborne pathogen.

While influenza takes its toll on thousands of elderly individuals worldwide, every year, pandemic influenza which occurred in 1918 caused the deaths of more than 20 million people mostly in their 20s and 30s.[15] This pandemic, while forgotten by many in the general public, has remained etched in the minds of public health and infectious disease experts all over the world. In 1976, when a single soldier died of swine flu in New Jersey and some of his compatriots came down with a milder version of the illness, a nationwide alert went into effect, millions were vaccinated, some with adverse effects but there was no pandemic. In 1997 when Avian influenza H5N1 struck Hongkong chicken markets,[16] 18 previously healthy young people were infected and six died (18%), a mortality rate much higher than the normal mortality rate for influenza. More than one million chickens were slaughtered and the disease was rapidly brought under control.

The World Health Organization recognized the efforts of the Hongkong authorities in averting a possible pandemic of influenza with a high mortality to which most humans were not immune. Sero-epidemiologic studies[17] of healthcare workers demonstrated the ability of the virus to be transmitted from person to person through direct contact, as individuals who reported bathing patients with avian influenza were at higher risk of sero-conversion. The serologic studies also demonstrated the efficacy of protective measures put in place at the time and the lack of efficient human to human transmission of the virus.[17]

It is against this backdrop of a recent novel avian influenza having emerged in southern China and a distant memory of a lethal pandemic which killed millions of young people that initial infection control measures directed against SARS need to be understood. In addition, SARS possessed an unusual quality in that it seemed to be far more efficiently transmitted in the healthcare setting than in households where measles, varicella and other airborne viruses usually rapidly took hold. This has yet to be explained completely but it buttresses the argument that close contact is the major mode of transmission of the SARS virus. It has been argued that Asian families have less close contact than healthcare workers and that this may be the reason for the differences in attack rates.

Nosocomial Viral Respiratory Infections

Nosocomial viral respiratory pathogens are not new. The literature is replete with reports of nosocomial transmission of pathogens that cause pneumonia.[18] In temperate countries, seasonal outbreaks of respiratory syncitial virus (RSV) cause a significant amount of morbidity and mortality in neonatal units and pediatric hematology-oncology units.[19] In staff, RSV is a major cause of sick leave in the winter months and many workers have investigated the efficacy of various methods aimed at preventing the nosocomial transmission of RSV. A four arm sequential trial[20] compared the effectiveness of cohort nursing alone, gloves, gowns and masks alone or a combination of cohort nursing, gloves, gowns and masks and found that either intervention alone (cohort nursing or personal protection) did not work in terms of reducing both transmission of the virus to sick children and infection of staff. On the other hand, a combination of cohort nursing and use of gloves, gowns and masks reduced the incidence of staff infections from 28% to 3%. Because of the morbidity associated with RSV, it is one of the best studied respiratory viruses.[19] Another well designed controlled clinical trial demonstrated the limitations of masks, gloves and gowns alone in preventing nosocomial transmission of RSV. A combination eye-nose mask which limited contact with HCW conjunctivae was more effective in reducing nosocomial spread of RSV than masks alone.[21] While RSV is a paramyxovirus, the modes of transmission by large particle droplets, close contact and probably fomites approximate those for the SARS coronavirus and we can probably extrapolate some of the science of SARS transmission from the lessons of the nosocomial epidemiology of RSV.

| Fomites have been a cause for concern with the SARS coronavirus since the initial global dissemination in the Hotel M to individuals who had no direct contact with the index case but stayed in the same corridor

Fomite Transmission

Other respiratory pathogens that have been transmitted by non-respiratory routes include the rhinoviruses that are causes of the common cold. In an elegant series of experiments designed by Dr Jack Gwaltney and his team at the University of Virginia, rhinoviruses were found to be efficiently transmitted through coffee cups and poker cards by individuals who were protected from large droplet aerosol transmissions.[22] (The role of fomites in the transmission of respiratory pathogens has always been the object of concern.[23] Smallpox is well known to be transmitted by fomites in addition to the well known airborne transmission by small particle aerosols. Indeed, one of the first well documented incidents of biological warfare was the use of smallpox infected blankets against Native Americans by the British commander Amerherst.[24]

Fomites have been a cause for concern with the SARS coronavirus since the initial global dissemination in the Hotel M to individuals who had no direct contact with the index case but stayed in the same corridor and probably had occasion to touch elevator buttons or railings which might have been contaminated by the SARS virus. With the Amoy Gardens outbreak in Hongkong,[25] more than 70 individuals who had no known direct contact were infected possibly through the aerosolization of contaminated sewage. The implications of fomite transmission of SARS are considerable. They would mandate a much greater degree of environmental cleaning than is considered reasonable if there is widespread dissemination of SARS in a particular area. There are many unanswered questions in this arena. For example, why did the individuals in the same hotel floor as the index case in Hotel M get infected but none of the staff?[7] In practical terms, the most logical infection control response to a disease which is well transmitted by fomites is to practice effective terminal disinfection in areas where individuals who are shedding the pathogen have come into contact. The use of gloves has also been shown to be highly effective in preventing the dissemination of vancomycin resistant enterococci, for example, without the addition of gowns.[26]

Coronaviruses and the Implications for Nosocomial Spread of SARS

SARS has been convincingly demonstrated to be caused by a coronavirus.[27] Nosocomial transmission of coronaviruses has been reported in the past. In a recent study from a Canadian neonatal and pediatric intensive care unit coronaviruses were found to be the commonest nosocomial viral infections[28] in the unit compared with RSV and influenza and adenoviruses which were the commonest causes of community acquired viral respiratory tract infections. Interestingly, the same study also found coronaviruses to be the most common viruses carried by staff working in the unit, although this was not consistently associated with symptomatic infection. Coronaviruses are best known as among the causes of the common cold. They are believed to be rare causes of lower respiratory tract infection because of their inability to proliferate efficiently at temperatures of 37C. Certain other characteristics of previously known coronaviruses 229E and OC43 are their ability to survive after drying on inanimate surfaces in the hospital environment as well as the differences in the viability of the virus at different conditions of temperature and humidity.[29,30] While the SARS coronavirus has a certain amount of homology with the other pathogenic human coronaviruses,[31] too little is known about its behavior under different environmental and atmospheric conditions to make a definitive statement about the role of the environment in nosocomial transmission. There have been reports, not yet in the peer reviewed literature, of the persistence of the SARS coronavirus for prolonged periods on environmental surfaces for up to two days.[32] Survival in stool is reported to be even longer — up to 4 days in alkaline diarrheal stools. This would certainly help to explain the circumstances such as the Hotel M outbreak.

SARS is a particularly virulent coronavirus because it is a novel coronavirus to which humans probably do not have any innate immunity. Individuals without any immunity when exposed to an airborne pathogen typically have very high attack rates with high fatality rates, for example, with measles and

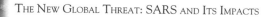

> **There have been reports, not yet in the peer reviewed literature, of the persistence of the SARS coronavirus for prolonged periods on environmental surfaces for up to two days.**

smallpox which decimated the native populations of the Americas. The relatively low attack rates documented with the SARS coronavirus would again argue against the airborne route as being a major mode of transmission. In Singapore for example, the index case for the national outbreak was nursed in a general ward by staff who were not wearing protection of any kind and the attack rate was only 1:8 doctors, 9:30 nurses and 1:12 fellow patients in the same ward areas.[33]

Infection Control for SARS: The Twin Pillars and Some Definitions

Infection control guidelines for SARS have focused on:

(1) personal protective equipment,
(2) quarantine and isolation or administrative and engineering controls.

These have been described as the two pillars of infection control for nosocomial respiratory pathogens with tuberculosis as the archetype of a nosocomial respiratory pathogen.

The following definitions are from the Hospital Infection Control Practices Advisory Committee of the US Centers for Disease Control and Prevention:[34]

Contact transmission could be either:

(a) Direct contact which involves the physical transfer of micro-organisms by body surface to body surface contact. Examples of diseases which are spread by direct contact include scabies or enteroviruses

(b) Indirect contact which involves an intermediate object usually

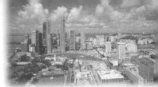

inanimate which has been referred to as a fomite. Examples of diseases which are well known to be spread through fomites include Clostridium difficile diarrhea.

Droplet transmission occurs when the source patient coughs or sneezes or generates a large respiratory droplet during a procedure such as suctioning or nebulizer therapy. Examples of diseases spread by droplets include mumps, rubella or meningococcal meningitis.

Airborne transmission refers to the spread of infectious agents by small particles, usually 5μ or smaller that can remain suspended in the air for longer periods of time and over longer distances. The major diseases spread by the airborne route include varicella, measles and tuberculosis.

Common vehicle transmission refers to transmission by contaminated items such as food, water or equipment. Cholera is the classic disease spread through a common source, usually water.

Tuberculosis as a Model for Infection Control for SARS

Tuberculosis is a disease known since the time of the Egyptians. Its contagion is also well known as the "White plague" which banished patients infected with tuberculosis to the Magic Mountain of Thomas Mann. Tuberculosis finally came under some form of control with the identification of Koch's bacillus and the development of diagnostic microscopy, cultures, therapeutics, skin testing and a vaccine which unfortunately has not proved as effective as was hoped. Rapid decreases in the incidence and mortality from tuberculosis

Droplet transmission occurs when the source patient coughs or sneezes or generates a large respiratory droplet during a procedure such as suctioning or nebulizer therapy.

251

> ## The transmission of SARS primarily to healthcare workers early in the course of the outbreak also resonated with those familiar with the history of tuberculosis.

were noted at the beginning of the 20th century in the US[35] and Europe as well as in the more developed parts of Asia such as Japan and Singapore. This was due to reforms in housing and sanitation and long preceded the development of streptomycin, the first effective anti-tuberculous drug that won Waksman the Nobel prize for medicine. In the 1980s and 1990s, outbreaks of nosocomial transmission of multi-drug resistant tuberculosis in healthcare workers[36] led to the proliferation of guidelines for tuberculosis prevention and control. In the US, the Federal Occupational Safety and Health Administration (OSHA) guidelines[37] include mandatory fit testing of employees which has had the unfortunate effect of turning infection control practitioners into what have been described as "facial hair police".[38] The emphasis on personal protective equipment has been seen by some as placing an undue emphasis on healthcare worker protection without consideration of the protection of, for example, other patients in the same area. The use of PPE is also not without its own adverse consequences[39] as reactions to latex are common among healthcare workers, some with serious consequences. It should also be noted that the use of respirators has been associated with fatal adverse events as well.[40]

Some of the lessons learned in the prevention of nosocomial transmission of tuberculosis can be applied to SARS. There is a considerable stigma associated with the disease as with tuberculosis which is sometimes described to this day in Singapore hospitals as "Koch's bacillus" so that patients will not hear the dreaded words "tuberculosis". It is ironic that the hospital which saw the initial widespread nosocomial transmission of SARS in Singapore[41] was Singapore's foremost tuberculosis hospital in the 1950s and 1960s when tuberculosis was highly prevalent in the city. Older healthcare workers could remember the association and were not surprised by the discrimination felt by healthcare workers from Tan Tock Seng Hospital. The transmission of SARS primarily to healthcare workers early in the course of the outbreak also resonated with those familiar with the history of tuberculosis. Medical historians record the invention of the stethoscope — that archetypal symbol of the physician — by Laennec so that he did not have to put his ear to the chest of a consumptive (tuberculous) patient and run the risk of contracting nosocomial tuberculosis. However, for all the parallels and the temptations to turn to the history books to prescribe protection for SARS, there remain major differences. The most important is the airborne transmission of tuberculosis. Although the evidence is not entirely convincing, there is data supporting the transmission of tuberculosis on occasion on airplanes.[42,43]

Airborne Viruses and Travel Restrictions

Other pathogens have also been documented to be transmitted on airplanes, most notably influenza.[44] On the other hand, despite all the WHO's restrictions on travel and their recommendations for airport screening, the number of individuals infected with SARS during air travel was remarkably low. According to the WHO,[45] there have been 35 flights carrying symptomatic probable SARS patients with 31 flights not resulting in a single secondary infection. Overall, 27 infections resulted from these individuals, One flight alone, CA112, which flew from Hong Kong to Beijing on 15 March, is now known to have accounted for 22 of the 27 cases. In Singapore, we had the experience of an individual who was so ill with SARS that she was transported straight from the airport to the hospital where she was promptly intubated and mechanically ventilated. Yet, in spite of that, no significant transmission on the plane was recorded despite active surveillance of all passengers on that flight. During the peak of the SARS epidemic in China, when the World Health Organisation had travel advisories and alerts in place, from 1 to 28 April 2003, there were more than 27,000 visitors from China and Hongkong[46] who entered Singapore with not a single recorded transmission from any of these individuals. In Taiwan, a strict 10-day quarantine[47] was placed on all individuals returning from countries which were on the WHO list of SARS affected countries. A total of 80,813 individuals were quarantined, out of which 11 had probable SARS and of these only one was laboratory confirmed SARS. Thus, the detection rate was 0.01% for probable SARS and 0.001% for laboratory confirmed SARS. This has to be balanced against the costs and psychological impact of quarantine for more than 80,000 individuals who were perfectly well. Most of the transmissions on airlines occurred in individuals seated near to the source, again supporting the contact and droplet transmission hypothesis. The furthest recorded transmissions occurred in passengers seven rows in front and five rows behind the source patient.[45] Travel restrictions seem to have had little impact in controlling the spread of SARS but they have crippled the economies of the worst hit countries, especially those which are highly dependent on tourism or international commerce such as Singapore and Hongkong. In the initial stages of the outbreak, when there was a great deal of uncertainty about the epidemiology of the virus and the disease appeared to be efficiently spread along international air travel routes, there might have been some justification for drastic recommendations to postpone "all but the most essential travel". Later, as the epidemic progressed and it became apparent that the infectivity was much lower than had been feared (in fact the rate at which the number of people were infected with each successive generation of the outbreak was progressively reaching extinction levels[48] in the SARS affected countries), it could be argued that WHO travel restrictions did a lot more harm than good by discouraging active case detection and by diverting resources away from the main centers of transmission of the virus — hospitals. One can only hope that if and when the virus reappears, perhaps in the Northern winter, that drastic travel restrictions are not instituted unless there is evidence of widespread dissemination of the virus across international air routes by travelers.

Engineering and Administrative Controls

All the guidelines agree that it would be ideal if patients with SARS can be nursed in isolation rooms.[8–13] There are differences in the recommendations

Most of the transmissions on airlines occurred in individuals seated near to the source, again supporting the contact and droplet transmission hypothesis.

There is a possibility that the virus might be aerosolized such as during high flow oxygen therapy or possibly even during the use of extractor fans

for negative pressure with separate ventilation systems and these perhaps reflect the differences in resources available for healthcare. One drawback of isolation rooms is that unless there are adequate nursing or medical resources, the degree of attention that the patient will receive in a single isolation room is obviously lower than in an open well ventilated area. In developed countries with mandated minimum nursing ratios, the use of single rooms with independent ventilation can be safely recommended without compromising patient safety, but there have been numerous anecdotal reports in Singapore and elsewhere of the dangers of keeping patients in single rooms out of the line of sight of the primary nurse caregivers in conditions of chronic nursing staffing shortages. Again, the mode of transmission plays an important role in deciding what degree of engineering and administrative controls are needed. If the virus is indeed airborne, then strict negative pressure needs to be maintained or else individuals exposed to exhaust air from patient rooms will be at risk of infection.

While all the evidence available points to droplet and contact transmission, there is a possibility that the virus might be aerosolized such as during high flow oxygen therapy or possibly even during the use of extractor fans which were blamed for the aerosolization of contaminated sewage during the Amoy Gardens outbreak.[25] N95 respirators or higher should be used. This is a cause for concern as in many countries without adequate pre-prepared negative pressure rooms, powerful extractor fans similar to the ones used in the bathrooms at the Amoy Gardens apartments are being used to create a form of laminar uni-directional airflow. While these may serve to direct the flow of air away from areas of heavy traffic, it is possible that they might be hazardous by causing the aerosolization of infectious droplets. There are other benefits to isolating patients with contagious diseases other than diverting their expired air away from others. These have been demonstrated in other nosocomial infections such as methicillin resistant *Staphylococcus aureus* (MRSA)[49] as well as other respiratory viral infections which are spread via the droplet route.[50] Madge *et al*. convincingly demonstrated, that for RSV, the archetypal nosocomial viral respiratory pathogen, cohort nursing when combined with use of PPE was highly effective in preventing transmission of RSV to both patients and staff.[20]

Isolation and Structural Issues

In Singapore[51] and Canada,[52] transmission of the SARS virus has been noted in crowded Emergency Rooms where patients routinely wait hours for a hospital bed. The waiting situation is common in emergency departments worldwide. In Singapore, SARS was documented as being transmitted to the visitor to a patient waiting in a corridor for a radiological procedure,[53] again a common occurrence in many healthcare settings. In our own hospital, the National University Hospital, the largest cluster of cases of SARS occurred in one of our "eight-bedded" wards[51] in which patients are deliberately placed eight to a cubicle in order to support the philosophy of healthcare financing in Singapore. The SARS outbreak has clearly been a wake-up call for health authorities worldwide[54] as they try to adjust health systems which have been primarily designed to minimize costs into systems designed to protect staff and patients. Often the adjustments are painful and costly.

The isolation and segregation of patients with suspect and probable SARS has been credited with markedly reducing the transmission of SARS.[48] (This is very likely to be true although with some viruses, most notably monkeypox,[55] the virus usually goes through a few generations then peters out due to repeated passage, which is the traditional approach to vaccine manufacture. Lipsitch

The SARS outbreak has clearly been a wake-up call for health authorities worldwide as they try to adjust health systems which have been primarily designed to minimize costs into systems designed to protect staff and patients.

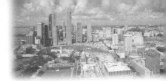

et al.[48] reported a reduction in time to isolation of patients with SARS as the epidemic progressed, as more was known about the virus and more strict measures were put in place.

Super Spreaders or Super Spreading Events?

The majority of individuals with SARS have not transmitted the virus to anyone.[53] While it is tempting to ascribe this to infection control measures, many of these individuals were infected and hospitalized long before the institution of infection control. This has given rise to the concept of "super spreaders". It is known that the presence of common viral upper respiratory tract infections can make some HCWs into "Cloud" healthcare workers.[56] These individuals have been linked with the airborne dispersal of agents which are normally only spread through contact such as Group A streptococci *or Staphylococcus aureus*. The hypothesis is that the presence of upper respiratory tract infections transforms these individuals into efficient transmitters of pathogens through an increase in the amount of coughing, sneezing or nose rubbing. Alternatively, airborne dispersal could result from the use of various respiratory therapies. The index case for the Singapore epidemic was not isolated and 22 HCWs, visitors and fellow patients were infected.[4] The second generation of cases associated with this cluster before the institution of infection control practices or strict isolation numbered only 13. The situation in Canada was similar with cases in the second generation pre-isolation.[57] It is quite clear, however, that non-isolated patients are hazardous to staff, visitors and other patients. Single non-isolated patients have led to well documented outbreaks in hospitals in Singapore,[51] Taiwan,[58] Canada[59] and Hongkong.[60] The phenomenon of "super spreaders" has been invoked to explain why so few transmissions resulted from the majority of non-isolated individuals while a few rare cases were associated with the vast majority of transmissions.[53] The jury is still out as to whether these are indeed individuals who are for some reason more able to transmit infection or whether events — such as the use of nebulizer therapy in an open crowded ward as had happened at the Prince of Wales Hospital in Hongkong[60] — are more responsible for what are probably more accurately described as "super spreading events". We await the publication of case control epidemiologic data to explain why some individuals in the

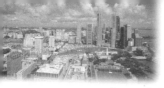

same cohort did not transmit the infection to anyone while others were associated with large clusters. Until such data are published, we have to assume that all individuals with SARS are "super spreaders" until proven otherwise and have to take all the necessary precautions.

Whom to Isolate?

Again because of the concern that an undiagnosed case might turn out to be a "super spreader", the threshold to isolation has progressively become lower. Initially, hospitals and clinics were using the World Health Organization case definitions of suspect and probable SARS cases to determine which cases to isolate. As we and others have pointed out, atypical presentations[61] are the Achilles heel of such a strategy and these have been associated with significant nosocomial transmission. In a very important paper from a SARS screening clinic, Rainer *et al.*[62] point out that the WHO criteria while relatively specific, have a sensitivity of only about 25% in predicting which individuals will turn out to have SARS. The implications are that a large number of individuals will need to be isolated and monitored very closely until their clinical course becomes evident. In practice in Singapore, this resulted in the conversion of large numbers of hospital wards to isolation facilities, cancellation of elective surgeries and an overall paralysis of the healthcare system. We used a regime of four hourly temperature monitoring without any use at all of anti-pyretics together with daily serial chest X-rays and blood counts and comprehensive chemistries. With such a regime, we found a sensitivity of 28%, specificity, 96%, positive predictive value, 11% and negative predictive value, 99% for the WHO criteria at presentation.[63] It is clear that we urgently need an accurate and rapid diagnostic test to allow us to filter out individuals who are at low risk of SARS, or better still at lower risk of transmitting the virus should they not be isolated. This has worked for the prevention of nosocomial RSV albeit imperfectly. In a study by Krasinski *et al.*,[64] a rapid screening protocol using an Enzyme linked Immunosorbent Assay, reduced the nosocomial transmission rate of RSV from 7.2 nosocomial infections per 1000 patient days to 0.5 infections per 1000 patient days. Unfortunately with SARS, the test will have to perform even better as a single non-isolated case could spell disaster.

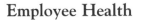

Employee Health

In developed countries, employee health programs are considered essential components of hospital infection control programs.[65] These programs are critical especially for diseases with prolonged incubation periods in which clusters of nosocomial infections in patients will not be manifested until patients are discharged or transferred to other hospitals or step-down care facilities where the clusters might not be recognized. Careful surveillance of ill staff has been instrumental in detecting outbreaks of diseases such as varicella[66] or measles.[67] With SARS, single infected HCWs who have continued to work due to staffing shortages have been connected with dozens of secondary cases in patients and fellow HCWs.[4] Most health systems in the 21st century are beset by chronic labor shortages and many staff feel under pressure to continue to work despite what they perceive to be minor illnesses. Human resource directors continue to view sickness absence as a negative point in job appraisals, further fuelling this practice which we now know can be lethal. There needs to be a major mindset change and perhaps a "most responsible staff" award can be given to the healthcare worker with the greatest number of sickness absences.

Fever Screening

Fever screening is widely practiced as a SARS-prevention measure. There was even a period when the World Health Organization called for fever screening at airports to prevent the global spread of SARS. There is no evidence that this did any good beyond further crippling the air travel industry.

Most health systems in the 21st century are beset by chronic labor shortages and many staff feel under pressure to continue to work despite what they perceive to be minor illnesses.

259

In fact, fever is a very non-specific and insensitive screening tool for SARS,[62] Atypical presentations of SARS without fever have been reported especially in older and immunocompromised patients.[61] One case is particularly illustrative[51] (Fig. 1): a 63-year-old man was cleared a fever triage area in an Emergency room as he was afebrile; he was then admitted to a general (not a "fever ward") ward as a case of heart failure and remained afebrile until he developed a low grade temperature after transfer to the Medical Intensive Care Unit for progressive shortness of breath. Two other patients, one visitor and one nurse in the same emergency department area were infected. The visitor, a previously healthy 28-year-old woman died and her husband and son were subsequently infected. In the brief period he was in the ward, two other patients and the entire shift of nurses working in the ward at the time who were only wearing N95 masks were infected. By the time he was febrile in the Intensive Care Unit, staff were wearing full PPE and no further infections resulted. Thus a single patient who "passed" two strict fever screens managed to be the source for at least nine infections in less than 24 hours. This patient was critically ill and died three days later and thus might have had a very high viral load.[25] This case illustrates the limitations of "cookbook screening" by using fever protocols without paying attention to a careful history and physical examination. In this case, the diagnosis was made by an alert cardiology team who re-did the history and examination and performed a bedside echocardiography to prove that he was suffering from pneumonia and not heart failure. Unfortunately, most health systems which attempt to be "cost-effective" would frown on clinicians who attempt to take too long to do a careful history and examination or to perform "high technology" investigations after office hours. This is one of the structural barriers which will need to be overcome for effective SARS infection control.

Interhospital Transfer of Patients

During the SARS outbreak, in Canada,[51] Taiwan[58] and Singapore,[53] the inter-hospital transfer of patients was a very efficient means of dissemination of the SARS virus. In Singapore, on March 22, the decision was made to close one hospital to new admissions to concentrate all SARS patients there.[41] This unfortunately led to patients recently discharged from this hospital being

During the SARS outbreak, in Canada, Taiwan and Singapore, the inter-hospital transfer of patients was a very efficient means of dissemination of the SARS virus.

shunted to other hospitals starting off epidemics there.[4] Now, in Singapore, once a cluster of cases with even a low degree of suspicion is identified, the unit is "locked down" with no admissions, transfers or discharges to prevent a recurrence of this situation. It is also the strategy used successfully in Vietnam to contain the virus, which led to Vietnam being the first country to be declared free of local transmission of SARS.[68]

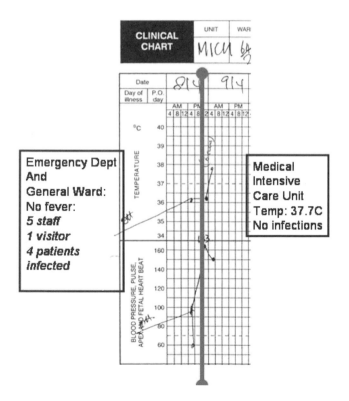

Fig. 1. Lack of sensitivity of fever screening for highly contagious SARS.

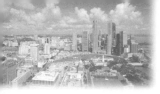

Personal Protective Equipment

Masks

The issue of whether N95 masks are adequate or whether N100 masks should be used in view of the size of the potentially infectious particle, was raised by a series of elegant experiments conducted by Singapore's Defence Science Organisation (unpublished data). There are practical considerations involved and N100 masks are very difficult to wear for prolonged periods of time. Like N95 masks, the costs associated with high filtration masks are considerable. In less well resourced environments, 12-ply cotton masks have been used and these have reportedly been effective in at least one large public hospital in preventing the nosocomial transmission of the virus.[69]

There is the concern that the use of N95 masks alone might not be adequate in the prevention of nosocomial transmission of SARS as cases have occurred in "fully protected" healthcare workers[70,71] possibly because of contact transmission. It is possible that surgical masks may be adequate for most exposures as has been suggested by Seto et al.[72] One alternative explanation for transmission of virus to fully protected individuals has been to blame the poor fit of the mask and advocate widespread fit testing. This has never been proved to be effective in the prevention of other airborne viruses despite the official sanction of the US Occupational Safety and Health Administration.[37] A more plausible hypothesis is that the SARS virus is transmitted primarily by contact and secondarily by large particle droplets. In that case, use of gloves for all contact with potentially infected surfaces and individuals is far more important than eliminating tiny leaks from masks or barring workers with unusual facial structures who are unable to pass "fit tests" from working with patients.

Gloves

Gloves have been demonstrated to be highly effective in the prevention of nosocomial infections, in particular pathogens which are known to persist on environmental surfaces such as *Clostridium difficile*[73] or vancomycin-resistant enterococci. The track record of gloves in the prevention of nosocomial viral infections is less well documented but they seem to be a logical, simple and practical method for protecting healthcare workers. Coronaviruses are known to persist on latex[29] and the use of gloves bypasses the natural antiseptic properties of human oils. This raises the important point that gloves need to be changed in between patients or else patients are at risk of infection from viruses carried on the gloved hands of healthcare workers. This has occurred early in the HIV era when HCWs were protected from bloodborne viruses by gloves but patients were infected by multi-resistant pathogens carried on the hands of healthcare workers.[34]

Gowns

Gowns have been widely used with little evidence because they are perceived to protect the clothes of the HCW. An important study by Slaughter et al.[26] showed that there was no difference between the use of gloves alone or gloves and gown in preventing the nosocomial transmission of multi-resistant bacteria. Gowns probably have a greater psychological impact as it is possibly easier to remember to wash your hands if you are removing a long sleeved gown.

Eye protection

Eye protection has been recommended by most authorities especially for aerosol generating procedures. However, the best data in support of the use of eye protection are from a pathogen transmitted by droplets. In a large controlled clinical trial, the use of eye-nose goggles[21] was associated with reduction in transmission of RSV that could not be achieved with masks alone. Case reports of transmission of SARS to healthcare workers wearing glasses, N95 masks, gowns and gloves have also given strength to this recommendation.[70,71]

Shoe covers and head covers

There is very little evidence in the literature and very little scientific data to support the use of shoe covers or head covers in the prevention of nosocomial

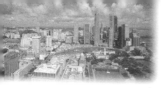

transmission of any of the well established nosocomial pathogens, let alone this novel pathogen and few would recommend their routine use.

Post-hospital

There are various recommendations for infection control for the handling of hospital wastes and the bodies of individuals who have died from SARS. While it is true that the virus can survive for some time outside of the body,[32] there is evidence that by the time patients become critically ill, their viral loads have actually dropped[25] and much of their illness is the result of an over-exuberant immune response. Thus the amount of live virus shed from a cadaver would be expected to be minimal. All the same, PPE should be worn by funeral workers and laboratory workers handling secretions from patients with SARS. It is noteworthy that for all the hundreds and probably thousands of HCWs infected with SARS during the epidemic, there were no well documented cases of infections in laboratory or autopsy staff.

Failure of PPE

While there have been reports of individuals who were infected while wearing full PPE, the details of adequate mask fitting, eye protection, etc. are not entirely clear. A single case from Taiwan[70] is instructive in which a physician using an N95 mask, double gloves and double gown while performing an ultrasound examination, was infected after spending a prolonged period at the patient's bedside. It is clear that we need to know a lot more about the virology of the SARS coronavirus before definitive recommendations can be made on PPE use.

Research Questions

While we have learned a tremendous amount in the brief period since SARS first emerged in November, there are a huge number of issues with importance for infection control in hospitals and healthcare facilities. I have a "wish list" of questions which I would like answered before we start preparing for the widely predicted and perhaps inevitable return of SARS:

1) Does airborne transmission of SARS ever occur? When? Can we safely restrict the use of N95 masks or higher to those situations?

2) Can we get a good test which allows us to rapidly detect early infection in patients with SARS?

3) What is the role of the environment? How frequently do we have to clean the bedrails of patients with SARS? Elevator buttons?

4) Are there asymptomatic carriers of the SARS coronavirus? Can they transmit infection? If asymptomatic individuals do not transmit infection, why do we quarantine them with punitive laws punishing quarantine breakers?

5) Is there such a thing as a super spreader? Is it genetically determined or is it due to a process such as nebulizer use which disseminates the virus?

6) How did the virus infect so many people at the Hotel M? Why were no other hotel clusters noted? What are the implications for international travel?

7) Is it possible to change the mindset of administrators to turn hospitals into places where people who are ill can be treated safely and efficiently rather than centers for profit to boost the economy?

Conclusion

I can only hope that the answers to these and numerous other questions raised by infection control practitioners, hospital epidemiologists, infectious disease clinicians and researchers can be answered before we face the next SARS outbreak or something worse! In July 2003, the best that we can offer is that SARS is caused by a coronavirus that appears to be efficiently spread in a healthcare environment especially by contact and by large particle droplets. Careful triage and isolation of potentially infected individuals and the use of masks (it is unclear which kind) and at least gloves is associated with a reduction in transmission. Full PPE alone, however, cannot completely eliminate transmission in certain settings probably associated with intense aerosolization of large numbers of viral particles from critically ill patients. While SARS shares the route of transmission of the common cold, RSV or mumps, it carries a mortality rate more than 100 times higher especially in older individuals with compromised immune systems, hence the urgent need to develop evidence based guidelines for prevention and control. While most healthcare systems will be able to handle typical cases with "classic" symptoms, atypical undiagnosed cases in our crowded wards and emergency rooms are potential hazards. Unless major structural changes are wrought in health systems across the world or alternatively a rapid test becomes available, we will most likely be very badly hit should the disease re-emerge in some rural community somewhere in East Asia next winter and spread across the globe again.

Glossary

Healthcare worker: Anyone working in a hospital environment, including doctors, nurses, allied health professionals, medical and nursing students, unit clerks etc.

Nosocomial infection: Arising from hospital. For patients, this is an infection which was not present or incubating at the time of admission; by convention, we use a cut off of 48–72 hours after admission to define an infection as nosocomial. For staff, it is an infection acquired in hospital and not in the community.

Pandemic: Infection that has spread over the whole world.

Contagious: Infection which spreads easily from person to person.

Sero-conversion: Blood test results were initially negative but later turned positive. This is usually used to indicate the development of antibodies by the immune system against the virus.

Morbidity: Illness.

Cohort nursing: Grouping patients with a particular condition together.

Fomite: Inanimate object which serves as an intermediate in the transmission of a microorganism.

Homology: Shared genetic or other characteristics.

Innate immunity: One we are born with.

Negative pressure room: One in which the air flows in one direction out of the room.

Passage of a virus: When a virus infects successive patients, i.e. from one to another.

References

1. Ksiazek T.G., Erdman D. and Goldsmith C., *et al.* A novel coronavirus associated with severe acute respiratory syndrome. *N. Engl. J. Med.* **348**: 1953–1966, 2003.

2. Drosten C., Gunther S. and Preiser W., *et al.* Identification of a novel coronavirus in patients with severe acute respiratory syndrome. *N. Engl. J. Med.* **348**: 1967–1976, 2003.

3. Lee N., Hui D. and Alan W., *et al.* A major outbreak of severe acute respiratory syndrome in Hong Kong. *N. Engl. J. Med.* **348**: 1986–1994, 2003.

4. Heng B.H. Epidemiology of SARS in Singapore. Tan Tock Seng Hospital *Medical Digest* 8–11, 34, 2003.

5. Booth C.M., Matukas L.M. and Tomlinson G.A., *et al.* Clinical features and short-term outcomes of 144 patients with SARS in the greater Toronto area. *JAMA* **289**: 2801–2809, 2003.

6. http://www.promedmail.org/pls/askus/f?p=2400:1001:529719 accessed 31 July 2003.

7. Centers for Disease Control and Prevention. Update: outbreak of severe acute respiratory syndrome — Worldwide. *MMWR Morb. Mortal Wkly. Rep.* **52**: 241–248, 2003.

8. http://www.who.int/csr/sars/infectioncontrol/en/ accessed 31 July 2003.

9. http://www.cdc.gov/ncidod/sars/ic.htm accessed 31 July 2003.

10. http://www.ha.org.hk/sars/ps/information/infection_control.htm accessed 31 July 2003.

11. http://www.hc-sc.gc.ca/pphb-dgspsp/sars-sras/prof_e.html accessed 31 July 2003.

12. http://www.gov.sg/moh/sars/information/healthcare.html#infectionctrl accessed 31 July 2003.

13. http://webjka.dph.gov.my/sars/guide.htm accessed 31 July 2003.

14. World Health Organisation. Influenza A H5N1 — Hongkong Special Administrative Region. *Weekly Epidem. Rec.* **78**: 49–50. 2003.

15. Luk J., Gross P. and Thompson W.W. Observations on mortality during the 1918 influenza pandemic. *Clin. Infect. Dis.* **33**: 1375–1378, 2001.

16. Yuen K.Y., Chan P.K.S. and Peiris M., *et al.* Clinical features and rapid viral diagnosis of human disease associated with avian influenza A H5N1 virus. *Lancet* **351**: 467–471, 1998.

17. Bridges C.B., Katz J.M. and Seto W.H., *et al.* Risk of influenza A (H5N1) among healthcare workers exposed to patients with influenza A (H5N1), Hong Kong. *J. Infect. Dis.* **181**: 344–348, 2000.

18. Musher D.M. How contagious are common respiratory infections? *New. Engl. J. Med.* **348**: 1256–1266, 2003.

19. Hall C.B., Douglas R.G., Geiman J.M. and Messner M.K. Nosocomial respiratory syncytial virus infections. *New. Engl. J. Med.* **293**: 1343–1346, 1975.

20. Madge P., Paton J.Y., McColl J.H. and Mackie P.L.K. Prospective controlled study of four infection-control procedures to prevent nosocomial infection with respiratory syncytial virus. *Lancet* **340**: 1079–1083, 1992.

21. Gala C.L., Hall C.B. and Schnabel K.C., *et al.* The use of eye-nose goggles to control nosocomial respiratory syncytial virus infection. *JAMA* **256**: 2706–2708, 1986.

22. Gwaltney J.M. and Hendley J.O. Transmission of experimental rhinovirus infection by contaminated surfaces. *Am. J. Epidemiol.* **116**: 828–833, 1982.

23. Hall C.B., Douglas R.G. and Geiman J.M. Possible transmission by fomites of respiratory syncytial virus. *J. Infect. Dis.* **141**: 98–102, 1980.

24. Stearn E.W. and Stearn A.E. *The Effect of Smallpox on the Destiny of the Amerindian.* Boston, Mass: Bruce Humphries; 1945.

25. Peiris J.S., Chu C.M. and Cheng V.C., *et al.* Clinical progression and viral load in a community outbreak of coronavirus-associated SARS pneumonia: a prospective study. *Lancet* **361**: 1767–1772, 2003.

26. Slaughter S., Hayden M.K. and Nathan C., *et al.* A comparison of the effect of universal use of gloves and gowns with that of glove use alone on acquisition of vancomycin-resistant enterococci in a medical intensive care unit. *Ann. Intern. Med.* **125**: 448–456, 1996.

27. Kuiken T., Fouchier R.A.M. and Schutten M., *et al.* Newly discovered coronavirus as the primary cause of severe acute respiratory syndrome. *Lancet* **362**: 263–270, 2003.

28. Gagneur A., Sizun J., Vallet S., Legrand M.C., Picard B. and Talbott P.J. Coronavirus-related nosocomial viral respiratory infections in a neonatal and pediatric intensive care unit: a prospective study. *J. Hosp. Infect.* **51**: 59–64, 2002.

29. Sizun J., Yu M.W.N. and Talbot P.J. Survival of human coronaviruses 229E and OC43 in suspension and after drying on surfaces: a possible source of hospital-acquired infections. *J. Hosp. Infect.* **46**: 55–60, 2000.

30. Ijaz M.K., Brunner A.H., Sattar S.A., Nair R.C. and Johnson-Lussenburg C.M. *J. Gen. Virol.* **66**: 2743–2748, 1985.

31. Ruan Y.J., Wei C.L. and Ling A.E., *et al*. Comparative full-length genome sequence analysis of 14 SARS coronavirus isolates and common mutations associated with putative origins of infection. *Lancet* **361**: 1779–1785, 2003.

32. http://www.who.int/csr/sars/survival_2003_05_04/en/index.html accessed 30 July 2003.

33. Hsu L.Y., Lee C.C. and Green J.A., *et al*. Severe acute respiratory syndrome (SARS) in Singapore: clinical features of index patient and initial contacts. *Emerg. Infect. Dis.* **9**: 713–717, 2003.

34. Garner J.S. Guideline for isolation precautions in hospitals. *Infect. Control Hosp. Epidemiol.* **17**: 53–80, 1996.

35. Centers for Disease Control and Prevention. Achievements in Public Health, 1900–1999: Control of Infectious Diseases, *MMWR Morb. Mortal Wkly. Rep.* **48**: 621–629, 1999.

36. Edlin B.R., Tokars J.I. and Grieco M.H. *et al*. An outbreak of multi-drug resistant tuberculosis among hospitalized patients with the acquired immunodeficiency syndrome. *N. Engl. J. Med.* **326**: 213–215, 1992.

37. US Department of Labor OSHA. Enforcement procedures and scheduling for occupational exposure to tuberculosis. OSHA Instruction CPL 2.106. Washington DC: Occupational Safety and Health Administration. pp. 1–21, 1996.

38. Blumberg H.M. Tuberculosis and Infection Control: What Now? *Infect. Control Hosp. Epidemiol.* **18**: 538–541, 1997.

39. Hunt L.W., Fransway A.F. and Reed C.E., *et al*. An epidemic of occupational allergy to latex involving healthcare workers. *J. Occup. Environ. Med.* **37**: 1204–1209, 1995.

40. Barach P., Rivkind A., Israeli A., Berdugo M. and Richter E.D. Emergency preparedness and response in Israel during the Gulf War. *Ann. Emerg. Med.* **32**: 224–233, 1998.

41. Chee Y.C. Severe acute respiratory syndrome (SARS) — 150 days on. *Ann. Acad. Med. Singapore* **32**: 277–280, 2003.

42. Kenyon T.A., Valway S.E., Ihle W.W., Onorato I.M. and Castro K.G. Transmission of multidrug-resistant Mycobacterium tuberculosis during a long airplane flight. *N. Engl. J. Med.* **334**: 933–938, 1996.

43. Centers for Disease Control. Exposure of passengers and flight crew to M. Tuberculosis on commercial aircraft: 1992–1995. *MMWR Morb. Mortal Wkly. Rep.* **44**: 137–140, 1995.

44. Moser M.R., Bender T.R., Margolis H.S., Noble G.R., Kendal A.P. and Ritter D.G. An outbreak of influenza aboard a commercial airliner. *Am. J. Epidemiol.* **110**: 1–6, 1979.

45. World Health Organisation. Global surveillance for Severe Acute Respiratory Syndrome. *Weekly Epidem. Rec.* **78**: 97–99, 2003.

46. http://www.cybrary.com.sg/pages/wkly28_04_03.pdf accessed 30 July 2003.

47. Centers for Disease Control and Prevention (CDC). Use of quarantine to prevent transmission of severe acute respiratory syndrome — Taiwan, 2003. *MMWR Morb. Mortal Wkly. Rep.* **52**: 680–683, 2003.

48. Lipsitch M., Cohen T. and Cooper B., *et al.* Transmission dynamics and control of severe acute respiratory syndrome. *Science* **300**: 1966–1970, 2003.

49. Shanson D.C., Johnstone D. and Midgley J. Control of a hospital outbreak of methicillin resistant Staphylococcus aureus infections: Value of an isolation unit. *J. Hosp. Infect.* **6**: 285–292, 1985.

50. Isaacs D., Dickson H., O'Callaghan C., Sheaves R., Winter A. and Moxon E.R. Handwashing and cohorting in prevention of hospital acquired infections with respiratory syncytial virus. *Arch. Dis. Child.* **66**: 227–231, 1991.

51. Fisher D.A., Chew M.H., Lim Y.T. and Tambyah P.A. Preventing local transmission of SARS: lessons from Singapore. *Med. J. Aust.* **178**: 555–558, 2003.

52. Dwosh H.A., Hong H.H.L., Austgarden D., Herman S. and Schabas R. Identification and containment of an outbreak of SARS in a community hospital. *Can. Med. Assn.* **168**: 1415–1420, 2003.

53. Centers for Disease Control and Prevention. Update: severe acute respiratory syndrome — Singapore, 2003. *MMWR Morb. Mortal Wkly. Rep.* **52**: 405–411, 2003.

54. Tambyah P.A. The SARS outbreak: How many reminders do we need? *Sing. Med. J.* **44**: 165–167, 2003.

55. Jezek Z., Grab B. and Dixon H. Stochastic model for interhuman spread of monkeypox. *Am. J. Epidemiol.* **126**: 1082–1092, 1987.

56. Sheretz R.J., Bassetti S. and Bassetti-Wyss B. "Cloud" health-care workers. *Emerg. Infect. Dis.* **7**: 241–244, 2001.

57. Poutanen S.M., Low D.E. and Henry B., *et al.* Identification of severe acute respiratory syndrome in Canada. *N. Engl. J. Med.* **348**: 1995–2005, 2003.

58. Centers for Disease Control and Prevention. Update: severe acute respiratory syndrome — Taiwan, 2003. *MMWR Morb. Mortal Wkly. Rep.* **52**: 461–466, 2003.

59. Centers for Disease Control and Prevention. Update: severe acute respiratory syndrome — Toronto, Canada, 2003. *MMWR Morb. Mortal Wkly. Rep.* **52**: 547–550, 2003.

60. Tomlinson B. and Cockram C. Sars experience at Prince of Wales Hospital, Hong Kong. *Lancet* **361**: 1486–1487, 2003.

61. Fisher D.A., Lim T.K., Lim Y.T., Singh K.S. and Tambyah P.A. Atypical presentations of SARS. *Lancet* **361**: 1740, 2003.

62. Rainer T.H., Cameron P.A., DeVilliers S., Ong K.L., Ng A.W.H., Chan D.P.N., Ahuja A.T., Chan Y.S. and Sung J.J.Y. Evaluation of WHO criteria for identifying patients with severe acute respiratory syndrome out of hospital. *BMJ* **326**: 1354–1358, 2003.

63. Tambyah P.A., Singh K.S., Habib A.G., Chia K.S. and Lim Y.T. Accuracy of WHO criteria for SARS in a non-SARS Singapore Hospital. *BMJ* in press.

64. Krasinski K., LaCouture R., Holzman R.S., Waithe E., Bank S. and Hanna B. Screening for respiratory syncytial virus and assignment to a cohort at admission to reduce nosocomial tranmission. *J. Pediatr.* **116**: 894–898, 1990.

65. Scheckler W.E., Brimhall D., Buck A.S., Farr B.M., Friedman C., Garibaldi R.A., Gross P.A., Harris J., Hierholzer W.J., Martone W.J., McDonald L.L. and Solomon S.L. Requirements for infrastructure and essential activities of infection control and epidemiology in hospitals: A consensus panel report. *Infect. Control Hosp. Epidemiol.* **19**: 114–124, 1998.

66. Raad I.I., Sheretz R.J. and Rains C.S., *et al.* The importance of nosocomial transmission of measles in the propagation of a community outbreak. *Infect. Control Hosp. Epidemiol.* **10**: 161–166, 1989.

67. Tambyah P.A., T.H.E. Tan, Lam W.C. and Lachai A.M. A nosocomial chickenpox outbreak related to herpes zoster in staff in a geriatric ward. In Program and Abstracts of the Forty-second Interscience Conference on Antimicrobial Agents and Chemotherapy, Chicago, IL, September 2002.

68. World Health Organisation. Vietnam — SARS free. *Wkly. Epidemiol. Rec.* **78**: 145–146, 2003.

69. Zhao Z., Zhang F., Xu M., Huang K., Zhong W., Cai W., Yin Z., Huang S., Deng Z., Wei M., Xiong J. and Hawkey P.M. Description and clinical treatment of an early outbreak of severe acute respiratory syndrome (SARS) in Guangzhou, PR China. *J. Med. Microbiol.* **52**: 715–720, 2003.

70. Twu S.J., Chen T.J. and Chen C.J., *et al.* Control measures for severe acute respiratory syndrome in Taiwan. *Emerg. Infect. Dis.* **9**: 718–720, 2003.

71. Centers for Disease Control and Prevention. Cluster of severe acute respiratory syndrome cases among protected healthcare workers — Toronto, Canada, April 2003. *MMWR Morb. Mortal Wkly. Rep.* **52**: 433–436, 2003.

72. Seto W.H., Tsang D. and Yung R.W., *et al.* Effectiveness of precautions against droplets and contact in prevention of nosocomial transmission of severe acute respiratory syndrome (SARS). *Lancet* **361**: 1519–1520, 2003.

73. Johnson S., Gerding D.N. and Olson M.M., *et al.* Prospective controlled study of vinyl glove use to interrupt Clostridium difficile nosocomial transmission. *Am. J. Med.* **88**: 137–140, 1990.

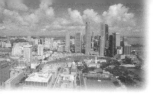

PAUL ANANTH TAMBYAH

Dr. Paul Ananth Tambyah is currently the Head of the Division of Infectious Diseases at the National University of Singapore. He is also Consultant Infectious Disease Physican at both the National University Hospital and Alexandra Hospital. He sits on numerous committees at the University and Ministry of Health, Singapore and is also currently President of the Society of Infectious Disease, Singapore. He is Chairman of the Scientific Committee for the 2nd Asia Pacific Conference on Infection Control and hopes you will attend the meeting now scheduled for March 2004. After completing his medical education in Singapore, he trained at the University of Wisconsin with Dr Dennis Maki. His main research interests are in catheter associated urinary tract infections and emerging infections in Southeast Asia, in particular the Nipah virus and the SARS coronavirus, and has published locally and internationally on these and other infectious disease subjects.

Associate Professor of Medicine
Consultant Infectious Disease Physician
National University of Singapore
Department of Medicine
5 Lower Kent Ridge Road
Singapore 119074
Tel: (65) 67795555
Fax: (65) 67794112
E-mail: mdcpat@nus.edu.sg

15

SARS — Lessons on the Role of Social Responsibility in Containing an Epidemic

by *Pheng-Soon Lee*

The World Health Organization and most doctors now accept that SARS first occurred in southern China in late November 2002. How this came about is uncertain, but it is possible that the infectious agent (now accepted as a new coronavirus and sometimes referred to as SARS-CoV) jumped the species barrier from animals to humans. (Scientists in China subsequently found evidence of this virus in three species of animals — palm civets, racoon dogs, and Chinese ferret badgers — that are sold alive in food markets. However, it is still unclear whether such animals, bred for human consumption, were the sources of the human outbreak.) In fact, rumors of an unusual febrile illness in Guangdong had been circulating for some time before the first cases appeared in Hanoi and Hong Kong, but there was no official confirmation of the outbreak or of any concerted governmental action within China.

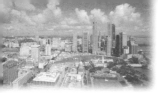

Epidemiologists have since worked out the sequence of events of this outbreak. In late February 2003, a single infected medical doctor from south China spent a single night on the ninth floor of a Kowloon hotel in Hong Kong. He infected at least 16 people either staying on, or visiting the same floor, and from this single event the international SARS epidemic began.

By March 12, 55 cases of SARS were recognized, mainly in hospitals in Hong Kong, Singapore and Hanoi. A month later, there were more than 3000 cases and 100 deaths in 20 countries worldwide. By May 8, 7000 cases, and by June 11, almost 8500 cases and more than 800 deaths, had been reported to the WHO from 29 countries. During the month of June, the number of new cases being reported had slowed down to a daily handful, and on June 19, marking the 100th day since the world was first alerted to the SARS epidemic, the WHO was speaking of this outbreak of SARS as being close to being defeated.

The SARS-CoV was conclusively identified as the cause of the epidemic on 17 April. However, to this day the disease remains without a vaccine, without effective treatment, and with a case-fatality rate of between 10 and 15%. The only possible measures against this outbreak were the centuries-old control measures used in epidemics before the age of antibiotics – isolation, contact-tracing and follow-up, quarantine, and travel restrictions. In our modern world, because of the speed of spread through international air travel, these measures had to be implemented on a monumental scale across the globe if there were to be any chance of containing the outbreak at all.

What has this Outbreak taught us about the Role of Social Responsibility?

SARS is not the only "new" epidemic, or indeed the "most fatal", of recent times. Around 30 such diseases have emerged during the past two decades or so, the most well-known being the Hanta virus and Ebola fever. The most deadly of these is probably Ebola, with some outbreaks reporting between 70 and 90% of infected cases dying. The most widespread of these is probably HIV-1, and today AIDS patients can probably be found in every country in the world. However, the epidemic with the greatest potential for spread is possibly SARS, and even if this current epidemic has since been controlled, there is no guarantee that another outbreak will not occur with the same devastating speed. This is because SARS has a relatively long incubation period of up to 10 days. This is more than enough time for any infected but apparently normal traveler, to literally circle the globe and carry the seed of a new epidemic to any country.

As scientific advances provide a better understanding of how the disease is transmitted, it offers the opportunity to protect both society and individuals through the modification of current social practices. In the early days of Ebola, the bodies of patients who died were prepared in the traditional way — by many members of the family participating in rituals of careful cleansing before burial. It was only when scientific findings showed that the Ebola virus was present in, and was transmissible through, the body fluids of the dead relatives, that such cleansing became much more limited, with the task being assigned to only one or two individuals carefully trained in personal hygiene. In another familiar example, when through scientific developments it was revealed that that HIV was transmitted through exposure to the body fluids of infected (but apparently normal) individuals, there was corresponding increase in awareness of the importance of social responsibility, in terms of modified the personal behavior of all individuals at risk, in controlling the disease. At the societal level, many countries provided clean syringes and needles to drug abusers in "exchange programs", thus avoiding the sharing of potentially infected needles. Sex workers were also educated about the need for insisting on the use of condoms during intercourse, and the words "protected sex" and "safe sex" crept into our vocabulary.

Similarly, we now understand how the new SARS virus is spread. The virus is known to be present in individuals for up to 10, and very occasionally more days, before the appearance of the first symptom — fever — and that transmission of infection by an infected person before the onset of fever is extremely rare. Detection of the first appearance of fever in at-risk individuals, is therefore critical. We also know now that this virus can be found in many body fluids, and microscopic droplets from the respiratory tract (e.g. resulting from sneezing, or from touching by an unwashed hand after contact with the nose and mouth) are a common way of dissemination. Practice of good personal hygiene by *everybody* is therefore also very important. On the other hand, it is also clear now that even if extreme care is exercised by an individual, unexpected routes of transmission can still "get to him", and therefore nobody is totally safe in an epidemic. In one of the better-studied outbreaks in

Hong Kong, it was concluded that the spread of droplets of infected fecal material, flushed down the toilet into the sewer pipe serving many apartments in one block, was the cause of transmission. Microscopic droplets of this infected material "vented backwards" into several apartments through dried out gully-traps in the floors of the bathrooms and infected many unsuspecting persons who were literally not safe in their own homes.

How has such knowledge changed our understanding of what constitutes "socially responsible behavior" in this "post-SARS" era? Can greater awareness of social responsibility help reduce the risk of spread, and perhaps even the risk of new outbreaks in the future? This question can be addressed at several levels.

First, on an International Level

SARS illustrated once again how an outbreak of a disease in one state can quickly spread throughout a country, then to neighboring countries, and finally around the world. The worldwide SARS epidemic began with just one person in a hotel room. Worldwide spread was possible because of two reasons. First, ignorance of the disease and its consequences at the individual level played a big role. Had the "index-case" doctor known more about the illness, might he have sought medical treatment earlier instead of traveling from China to Hong Kong, and if his doctors had known more about the illness when they first saw him, might they have taken more stringent efforts to isolate him from the start? During the early stages of the epidemic, however, very few people had any knowledge of the disease. Second, the window-period of up to 10 days during which an infected person feels totally normal, combined with the ease of air-travel, means that an infected person could literally be on the other side of the globe before he realized something was wrong. Doctors in yet-unaffected countries therefore need to have access to good information of epidemics anywhere in the world delivered to them in a timely manner.

Therefore, the development and application of good health surveillance and reporting systems, careful monitoring of health statistics and early follow-up of unexplained illness and death, and early notification of International bodies like the WHO, are very important. The safety of the whole world depends on high standards of these public health measures being practiced in all countries. Moreover, excluding specific countries from international

On an international level, therefore, social responsibility includes open collaboration between countries as well as honesty across borders.

participation in health forums (e.g. Taiwan from WHO meetings) for political reasons hurts many countries apart from the one being targeted. On an international level, therefore, social responsibility includes open collaboration between countries as well as honesty across borders.

Second, at an Institutional (e.g. hospital) Level

The SARS outbreak required that all febrile patients be kept in separate, well-ventilated facilities. In Singapore, febrile patients with either a history or clinical signs adequate to make them suspect SARS cases, were sent to a designated hospital (Tan Tock Seng Hospital) with the necessary facilities manned by well-trained, battle-experienced staff. Not only were the movement of staff and patients between hospitals (e.g. for specialist tests or to use facilities available only in one location) kept to a minimum, but also all healthcare professionals had to be extremely careful with infection-control procedures (including use of respirators, gowns and gloves in higher-risk areas however uncomfortable these were in practice) when attending to patients.

In addition, the number of visitors to hospitals had to be minimized to reduce the risk of introducing the infection to the general community from the affected hospital. In the same light, two events in the last epidemic come immediately to mind. The first was the way in which all the staff in the one affected hospital in Hanoi decided to isolate themselves in the hospital till the disease burnt itself out, claiming several of them, but thereby sparing the community. The second was the way in which a young vascular surgeon in the Singapore General Hospital, realizing that he was febrile and therefore probably infected with SARS, drove past his home waving farewell to his children from his car, in his final journey to the hospital to check himself in for treatment. SARS claimed him, but left his family untouched.

All the staff in the one affected hospital in Hanoi decided to isolate themselves in the hospital till the disease burnt itself out, claiming several of them, but thereby sparing the community.

SARS required even lower-risk institutions to exercise extra care. In Singapore, the Ministry of Health applied very stringent mandatory measures for all clinics, even those of lower-risk general practitioners (GPs). These included the early assessment of patients with a higher risk of SARS (by requiring all patients to declare any travel history and any contact with possible SARS patients, as well as by checking their body temperature immediately upon arrival to the clinic). Febrile and other higher-risk patients were given masks and instructed to keep within a designated segregation area. Great care was paid to the log book maintained in each clinic — details like the time physically spent by patients on the premises were recorded to allow contact-tracing, should any patient seen that day be later confirmed as SARS-infected. Voluntary actions taken by socially responsible GPs included stopping their medical practice immediately upon being notified that a patient that they had recently seen was confirmed as a case of SARS- until after a self-imposed quarantine period of 10 days was over. These measures may have paid off handsomely for Singapore — nobody was infected by SARS simply by having shared the same waiting room of a GP's clinic with another patient later confirmed to have SARS.

These important measures were imposed in non-medical institutions as well. In Singapore, visitors to many buildings, and certainly to all government offices, could enter only after signing a declaration of no-travel to SARS affected countries, and after having had their temperatures checked. In time, "ear thermometers" were replaced by non-intrusive walk-through thermal scanners located at building entrances. Well after the outbreak of SARS has ended, all incoming passengers in Singapore's Changi International Airport are still being scanned for fever. During the epidemic, even outgoing patients were scanned - an example of social responsibility being practiced by a country unwilling to "export" cases of SARS — even of transit passengers — to its neighbors.

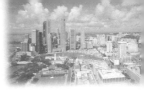

Finally, at the Personal level

It is here that social responsibility can make the greatest difference.

a) Greater care about our own personal movements will enable us to remember if we have been to a place subsequently found to have been visited by an infected person. In Singapore during the epidemic, this came down to noting fine details, even of the date, time and registration number of a taxicab that one took.

b) In China and many other countries, spitting in public places has changed from being just a filthy habit, to an offence punishable by law. Even now, months after the last case of SARS, a person can draw undue attention to himself merely by sneezing loudly in public.

c) Wearing of masks in public (common in Hong Kong and south China during the period of maximal outbreak) is no longer seen. However, other personal protection measures like careful hand-washing before eating, and greater responsibility for personal hygiene, have become commonplace, the benefit of well-conducted mass-education campaigns.

d) Self-monitoring of body temperature at home used to be common during the epidemic, and employees were encouraged to stay away from work if they had a fever, however slight, with instructions to seek early medical assistance if the fever persisted. This is now no longer commonplace, but many doctors sense that their patients still seek treatment earlier if they have a fever from any cause.

e) The Chinese habit of helping oneself to food from a communal plate, using one's own chopsticks, has since been replaced by compulsory use of serving spoons. Hopefully, this good habit is here to stay.

f) During the SARS epidemic in Singapore, even funeral rites were changed. Known and suspect SARS patients who passed away in hospitals would first be sent for post-mortem examination, and then their remains would be hermetically sealed twice in strong black plastic bags before being enclosed in a coffin. Cremation had to be carried out within 24 hours, without the benefit of a prolonged wake as was traditionally practiced. Because of sensitivity to religious practices, Muslim patients could be buried rather than be cremated, but their bodies were brought directly from the hospital to the cemetery rather than to the home first for a wake. Though these practices have since stopped, they served to show citizens that in times of crisis, important personal sacrifices like forgoing a "proper" funeral for loved ones would have to be made.

At the time of writing, the current SARS epidemic is over. Even so, many measures first started as personal social responsibility, particularly those revolving around good personal hygiene, are still being encouraged by social campaigns in several countries. Similarly, many countries that have installed walk-through thermal scanners in key locations (e.g. hospitals, airports, governmental buildings) still have them in place. Most authorities do not discount the possibility that SARS may recur during the next winter, and measures of social responsibility so carefully cultivated this recent past, should not be discarded so readily.

Social Irresponsibility

For completeness sake, it is important to record that social responsibility during the epidemic had not always been easy to achieve. For example, during the earlier stages of the outbreak in Taiwan, scenes of loudly protesting healthcare workers, angry at being quarantined within their hospitals, were broadcast on TV in many countries. In Hong Kong, health officials moving into the affected Amoy Gardens complex of apartments to impose quarantine after a large cluster of cases had occurred in one block, found that many of the residents

Most authorities do not discount the possibility that SARS may recur during the next winter, and measures of social responsibility so carefully cultivated this recent past, should not be discarded so readily.

had simply left without word, and did not return for contact tracing even when publicly urged to do so. In Singapore, a family identified at one GP's clinic as being possible SARS patients, ignored instructions to wait for the assigned ambulance to arrive to bring them to the designated hospital. Instead, they wandered around the neighborhood shops, even though they almost certainly knew the hazard they posed to others by so doing. And also in Singapore, the authorities found that home quarantine orders sometimes had to be supplemented by the force of law and the deterrence of punishment, to ensure that all people exposed to the risk of SARS stayed at home till they could be confirmed as uninfected at the end of an incubation period.

Conclusions

When the SARS epidemic first started, many people thought of it purely as a medical problem. The expectation was that doctors and scientists would identify the cause, find a cure, and treat the sick. However, because the disease spread so rapidly, especially among care-givers like hospital staff, it quickly became recognized as a disease that would change the way medicine was practiced — i.e. extreme care had to be taken to prevent self- and cross-contamination. It was also recognized as a terrible danger to all of society.

All the affected countries have now been declared SARS-free. However, the experience in each has shown clearly that SARS is an epidemic that requires the cooperation of health-care workers and lay citizens to overcome it, and more important, to help reduce its spread should it recur. This is important because even though the virus causing it has been identified, there is still no cure, no vaccine, and no means of reducing the mortality rate. In dealing with future outbreaks of this disease, we will still have to rely on the time-honored methods of epidemic control, namely, isolation, contact-tracing and follow-up, quarantine, and travel restrictions, and success in these measures requires the full cooperation of all citizens.

This outbreak has therefore modified not just how doctors look at medicine and its practice, but also confirmed how much society needs to rely on social responsibility at all levels in epidemic control. These costly lessons will surely enable a swifter, more effective response in any future epidemics — whether caused by a recurrence of SARS or a new disease.

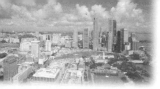

PHENG-SOON LEE

Dr. Pheng-Soon Lee, BSc (Hons), MBBS, FFPM, MBA, is currently President of the Singapore Medical Association and Honorary Fellow, Department of Human Nutrition, Otago University NZ. He is the Regional Medical Director, Mead Johnson Nutritionals.

Correspondence to: Dr. Pheng Soon Lee, E-mail: lee_ps@pacific.net.sg.

16

Combating SARS with Infrared Fever Screening System (IFss)

by *Yang How Tan*

Summary

When Severe Acute Respiratory Syndrome (SARS) hit Singapore, one key factor in containing its spread was the early detection of probable SARS cases. When it was found that one of the earliest detectable symptoms was fever, it was imperative that we find a way to screen large groups of people quickly and non-intrusively for fever. A team of defence engineers led by the Defence Science & Technology Agency (DSTA), an agency of the Singapore

283

government[a], quickly identified the thermal-imaging sensor used in the military as a possible device for such temperature screening. Relevant software and hardware were added to the sensor and the Infrared Fever Screening System (IFss) was developed. Validation and reliability tests were conducted and the IFss was carefully calibrated for more accurate reading of skin temperature. It was proven to be effective as the first line of screening as it could scan a large number of passengers within a short time. Passengers with a high temperature would be directed to undergo temperature check with the use of an oral thermometer. The system was subsequently deployed at the various air, land and sea checkpoints. The development of the IFss demonstrated the defence community's ability to swiftly mobilize and respond quickly to deliver an innovative solution to fight against SARS . The IFss attracted a string of compliments from the media worldwide and contributed greatly to the government's efforts in boosting the level of confidence in Singapore among foreigners and locals.

Introduction

When the World Health Organization (WHO) issued a global alert and called for all air passengers to be screened in March 2003, SARS-affected areas including Canada, Hong Kong, Singapore, Vietnam and Guangdong province in China were advised to put in place some precautionary measures. Singapore implemented a range of measures. Several nurses and paramedics were stationed at our airport to conduct health screening of passengers arriving at Singapore Changi Airport from SARS-hit countries. Health declaration forms were introduced for all arriving and departing passengers. Unnecessary travel to SARS-affected areas was strongly discouraged.

However, the SARS virus continued to spread around the world. By 2 April 2003, WHO reported that SARS had affected some 17 countries and had taken the lives of several hundreds of victims. There was heightened concern over the import of SARS cases and the spread of the virus across borders.

---

[a] DSTA is the national authority for defence science and technology. We acquire, upgrade, design and develop systems to meet the defence and security needs of Singapore.

We identified the thermal imager as a highly possible device for such temperature screening.

Operational Limitations

In Singapore, more than 100 nurses and paramedics were stationed at the Singapore Changi Airport to spot incoming passengers who were unwell and checked their temperatures using oral or ear thermometers. Passengers with a temperature above 38°C were then sent to the Tan Tock Seng Hospital which was the designated hospital for SARS treatment for further medical assessment to see if they had symptoms of SARS .

Similar screening measures were also put in place at the Singapore Cruise Centre to screen incoming sea passengers from SARS-affected countries.

However, the conventional method of taking oral/ear temperatures of passengers suspected to have fever was time consuming and posed inconvenience to passengers during disembarkation. On average, it took six to eight nurses more than 15 minutes to screen one flight of some 150 passengers. Passengers also had to pass through a phalanx of inquisitive nurses in their protective gowns and masks upon their arrival. It was relatively quite unpleasant for visitors to Singapore.

The need to deploy nurses to these checkpoints added more strain on the demand for nurses, who were already stretched coping with their work at the various hospitals.

When the Ministry of Health (MOH) approached DSTA in the morning of 3 April 2003 to help provide possible screening devices that could be deployed to identify possible SARS cases, I met up with our Electro-Optics Programme Manager, Mr Teo Chee Wah at DSTA's Sensor Systems Division. We understood the urgency of having a fever screening system operational within the shortest time possible. Our expertise in systems engineering and integration enabled us to approach the existing viral outbreak from a holistic perspective, and to devise a systematic solution to the problem. We brainstormed on various possible solutions, with a focus on tapping existing resources so as to quickly deliver a device to meet the urgent need.

We identified the thermal imager as a highly possible device for such temperature screening. Such thermal imaging sensors are used commonly by the military forces, especially those in developed countries. Basically, the thermal imagers sense heat that is generated by an object — it can be a tank, a car, a person or even an animal. As long as heat is generated, the sensor will be able to pick up the heat and map the image of the subject. And we had delivered several of such thermal imagers to the Singapore Armed Forces (SAF) just a few years back. Back then, we worked with the SAF planners in jointly developing the operational and technical requirements, and contracted our strategic industry partner, Singapore Technologies (ST) Electronics to develop and manufacture the sensors that meet the SAF's unique operational requirements. The sensors are currently used with the operational weapon systems to enable the systems to operate at night.

With the birth of the idea of adapting a thermal imaging sensor, we proceeded to find out more about body and skin temperatures and explore how feverish persons could be diagnosed more accurately with the use of sensors. I leveraged on the network of domain experts within DSTA, DMRI (Defence Medical Research Institute) and DSO National Laboratories, to seek input and ideas on using an infrared sensor for skin temperature sensing and pertinent issues related to human physiology. Chee Wah and I put off all our other duties and focused our total energy to tackling this extremely urgent and important task. We met up with officials and medical doctors from MOH in the afternoon of the same day to understand the requirements in greater detail as well as to listen to other ideas and views gathered by MOH.

Fundamental Considerations

The WHO and the Communicable Disease Centre guidelines established that a suspect SARS case has a body temperature greater than 38°C. Therefore, the key performance objective of the device is to be able to identify with high confidence any probable fever cases so that screening could be done quickly. Those with a higher-than-normal temperature would then go through a more thorough medical assessment.

The military cooled thermal imager is a very sensitive and efficient piece of equipment, which can detect relative temperature differences of a distant

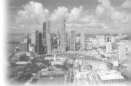

We worked on the hypothesis that infrared radiation from the skin could be used to estimate skin temperature and an elevated skin temperature is a proxy indication of core body temperature

object against a cooler background. Unlike a conventional thermometer, it was not designed to measure absolute temperatures. So the ideal device has to be carefully calibrated in real time to ensure a more accurate sensing of the temperature of any object in the field of view without any physical contact.

Human physiology

We worked on the hypothesis that infrared radiation from the skin could be used to estimate skin temperature and an elevated skin temperature is a proxy indication of core body temperature under some controlled environment and physiological condition. Research that has been done showed that human beings have a core body temperature which ranges from 36–38°C. The body naturally develops many mechanisms to regulate its core body temperature within the range of 36–38°C. One of mechanisms is radiating heat from the skin. When a person runs a fever, his/her skin temperature would be typically expected to rise. Skin temperature can thus be used as an indirect indicator of the core body temperature.

We consulted our fellow colleagues in DSTA's Defence Medical Research Institute (DMRI) and search the medical literature on the web for useful and relevant information to complement what we had already known from our military sensor development work over the years. We learnt that skin temperature of a normal person ranges between 32–36°C. Skin temperature, unlike the core body temperature, varied at different parts of the body. It is also subjected to both internal environment (such as after an exercise or change in hormones, such as adrenaline) and external environment (such as the ambient temperature). And skin temperature on the face (i.e. forehead, face and neck) differs significantly between normal and feverish individuals. This

287

is indeed our own experience — as parents we use our palm [or the backside of the palm] to sense the temperature of the face of our children when we suspect that they are having a fever — before we bring them to see a family doctor. This temperature change and distribution is observable externally to deduce that a person is running a higher-than-normal temperature. Hence the thermal imager can be used to detect such differences in temperature.

We then worked with several assumptions based on the initial requirements of screening air passengers. Research on human body thermography has shown that skin IR radiation of a normal population, at resting metabolic rate and with normal clothing in a room temperature of 15–20°C, corresponds to a mean skin temperature of 32–35°C. As movement onboard an airplane is restricted and the environment is controlled, i.e. it is air-conditioned, the body metabolic rate of the arriving passengers will generally be close to that of the resting metabolic rate. Passengers with a fever would likely demonstrate a similar distribution of their skin temperature, but with a higher mean temperature.

We also decided to focus the reading of the skin temperature on the forehead and neck, as these selected facial regions have a narrow layer of tissue and reading the temperature could be made readily.

Based on our expertise and experience in military surveillance radar, we drew an analogy between the massive passenger fevers screening operation at the arriving aerobridge in Changi Airport to that of a radar detection environment. In general, air defence radar will scan its radar beam continuously and search a large surveillance space for potential targets. There are actually very few real targets of interest in the huge air space, but the radar processor has efficiently searched for them, and detect and track the real targets. The overall design of the radar system will determine its effectiveness and efficiency. We came across a proven technique in the radar signal detection and processing, commonly known as double-threshold detection approach. We adopted this approach to the fever screening issue.

The two levels of thresholds were identified as:

First tier — to use a system including a thermal imager to rapidly scan and screen a larger pool of passengers efficiently as they pass through the device. Passengers detected to have a higher-than-normal facial skin temperature are assumed to have a higher body core temperature. These passengers will thus

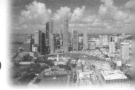
be led to undergo a second stage of screening to assess if they were indeed running a fever.

Second tier — experienced nurses equipped with the oral thermometer will further assess if the passengers are running fever and note if they have other SARS symptoms.

The device has to be calibrated to ensure unbiased sensing of the true skin infrared energy. According to Planck's Law, all objects with temperatures above absolute zero, i.e. 0 Kelvin, emit infrared (IR) radiation, and there is correlation between IR radiation energy and temperature. As can be seen in Fig. 1, the higher the temperature, the higher the IR energy radiated by an object at a particular electromagnetic wavelength. Since the human body temperature is about 300K, the skin will have a maximum IR energy radiation at a wavelength of around 10-micrometer.

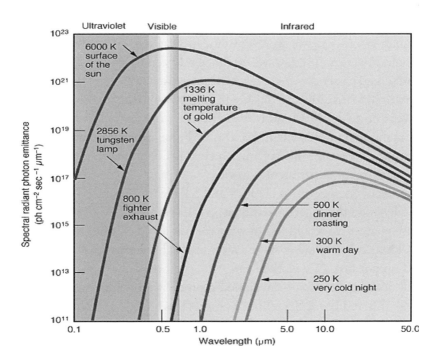

Fig. 1. Energy versus wavelength for various temperatures.

A thermal imager can capture this energy as it is made up of many small detectors (infrared radiation sensitive materials bonded on electronic read-out chip). The proposed sensing system would use a thermal imager to sample the IR energy radiated from a scene at a very high refresh rate and generates a video image to map and display the energy.

A thermal reference source (TRS) serving as a constant and stable thermal energy source is another key component. IR energy radiated from all objects in the sensor's field of view can be compared with the IR energy radiated from the TRS. When the IR energy radiated by the object (be it parts of a human body or other objects in the background) is higher than that from the TRS, the image of the object will display red. The temperature of the TRS thus allows more accurate temperature threshold setting.

A Prototype of the IFss

After much discussion, we were convinced that the thermal imager, with additional software and hardware, could be adapted to work as a temperature device to screen passengers for fever. However, there were a series of questions which we need to investigate to ensure the effectiveness of the proposed system. So we went on to develop a prototype and carry out further investigations.

As the thermal imagers belong to the SAF, we approached and shared our plans with the Defence Ministry and successfully obtained a set of the sensors to proceed with our experimental work.

Our team of engineers from DSTA and ST Electronics raced against time, as we understood the urgent need to stop the spread of SARS . We all knew the consequences we would face if we were not able to bring the virus under control. Human lives were at stake. We were highly motivated and remained focussed on our task. We worked into the wee hours of the morning and in less than 36 hours, we have developed a prototype of the system which we named — Infrared Fever Screening System (IFss).

A complete setup of the IFss is shown in Fig. 2. It consists of a thermal imager, a TRS, a central processing unit (CPU) and display monitors. The thermal imager captures IR energy from the scene, which is converted to electrical signals that are processed by the CPU for display on the flat-screen monitors.

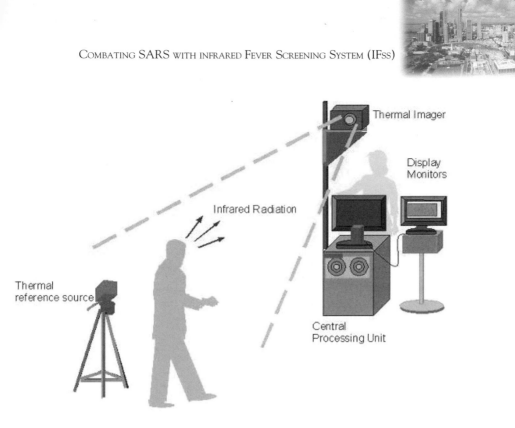

Fig. 2. A complete set-up of Ifss.

When a passenger passes through the sensor, the level of his skin IR radiation is unobtrusively detected and compared against the calibration instrument; the thermal reference source. There is no need for the passenger to stop. The face and neck regions of the passenger will appear in the field of view of the thermal imager as he walks pass the thermal reference source. Radiation energy captured by the thermal imager will be fed into a computer CPU. As shown in Fig. 3, feverish foreheads will show up as red spots and cool ones as yellowish-green/blue — on silhouetted images on the flat-screen monitor. The whole process takes less than a second. The operator, once trained, can view the display monitor and easily spot passengers with higher-than-normal temperature just by looking at the percentage and size of the red patches displayed on the face and neck. Those passengers with a high temperature will then be channeled to a more thorough medical assessment by the nurses.

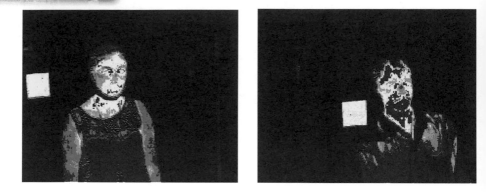

Fig. 3. IFss images

System Performance

We noted that the performance of the IFss is highly dependent on some key parameters including the settings of the thermal imager, the threshold settings of the TRS and consistency in the surrounding environment. Technical parameters of a thermal imager include uniformity, drift, minimum detectable temperature difference (affected by number of quantization levels, uniformity, max drift between self corrections), distance effect, as well as accuracy and stability of the TRS must be specified accurately so as to ensure the robustness of the system.

The IFss was to be installed in an environment which demonstrated consistency in temperature, preferably in an air-con environment. In addition, the IFss should not be set up facing glass panels, or directly under air-con outlets or halogen lamps. These could affect accurate reading of the temperature.

Trial Tests

A series of trial tests were subsequently conducted to verify the effectiveness of the IFss which we have developed, and to obtain a suitable set of threshold settings.

Trials were first conducted at the Accident & Emergency (A&E) Department of the Singapore General Hospital on 4 April. The main aim was to calibrate the thermal imager and study the characteristics of average skin temperatures of feverish patients. Skin temperature observed was generally a couple of degrees Celsius lower than core temperature. Therefore, the threshold setting of the TRS had to be set lower than 38°C. Considerations were made to ensure setting of the threshold will minimize the number of false alarms and misses. We decided to calibrate the system very conservatively to ensure that even those with the slightest doubt will be directed for further checks. So the chances of passengers with fever slipping through are quite unlikely.

The prototype was calibrated accordingly and temperatures of patients were recorded and verified against their temperature reading from oral thermometer. Results obtained from the trial were shown to doctors, nurses and MOH officials. We were confident of concluding that the IFss was effective in sieving out patients with core body temperature higher than 38°C.

Similar trials were then conducted using the prototype at a military medical center and workflow demonstration was carried out at the Singapore Changi Airport on 7 April 2003.

More trials were conducted on more selected flights in the following few days. Nurses, using ear thermometers, measured core body temperature of every passenger on selected flights. Data collected were validated to verify if there were any misses and those detected by the IFss had indeed higher-than-normal body temperature. The results proved very positive. When we presented our system solution and research findings to the MOH and other relevant authorities, a decision was made to deploy more sets of the IFss at the airport. The IFss was officially declared operational at Changi Airport on 11 April 2003.

While some members of the team continued to draw more sets of the military thermal imagers from the Defence Ministry and worked to deliver more sets of the IFss in the shortest time possible, another group of us carried out more trial tests. Two more trials were conducted — one at the Dieppe Barrack Military Camp and the other at the A&E Department of the Alexandra Hospital — to obtain the optimal threshold settings.

From the test results, we concluded that the mean skin temperature of a normal population observed to be similar to those found in the open literature. The mean forehead skin temperature of 36 adults at rest condition was found to be 32.85°C, with a standard deviation of 0.95°C. Therefore the probability of a normal person having a forehead skin temperature below 34.75°C (2σ above mean) is 97.5%. This result reaffirmed the false positive performance of our initial threshold setting we had set for the IFss.

Data obtained at the Alexandra Hospital was analyzed and it was noted that the IFSS had successfully spotted all test cases of patients with a body core temperature above 38°C.

With the establishment of the appropriate threshold settings, the IFSS has proved to be highly efficient and effective in detecting people with a higher-than-normal temperature for a second manual temperature check.

Deployment of the Fever Scanners

The IFss has made it practicable for us to screen large groups of people coming into as well as going out of Singapore, and to do this efficiently, effectively and very importantly, unobtrusively. Passengers no longer need to stop for temperature checks. A flight of passengers could be screened in a much friendlier way, as compared with a line of nurses, and almost instantaneously. By 15 May, of the tens of thousands of passengers screened at the airport, about 1548 were referred to medical staff for further examination. Fifty of them were subsequently sent to TTSH for medical examinations. It would have been impractical for the nurses to screen the same number of passengers without the IFss. The IFss has enabled more than 100 nurses to be re-deployed to the hospitals where they were urgently needed. In the weeks that followed, more sets of the IFss were deployed at all Singapore's air, land and sea checkpoints. At the height of the crisis, our government also loaned some sets of the IFss to Toronto, Hong Kong, Beijing and Taipei to help these SARS-hit countries in their efforts to curb the epidemic. Figure 4 shows the IFss in operation at the Woodlands checkpoint.

The development of the IFss sparked interests worldwide. We received many enquires from various authorities and organizations locally and abroad. Many have expressed interest in purchasing the system. Several companies,

> **At the height of the crisis, our government also loaned some sets of the IFss to Toronto, Hong Kong, Beijing and Taipei to help these SARS-hit countries.**

including ST Electronics, started marketing similar systems using the commercially available thermal imaging cameras. A patent for the IFss was filed. A national technical committee was set up and a Singapore Technical Reference was drawn up to help evaluate and ensure commercial scanners meet appropriate standards for mass fever screening.

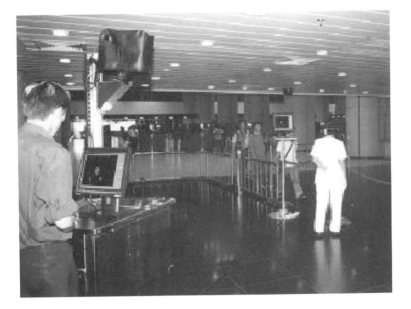

Fig. 4. IFSS in operation.

Conclusion

The IFSS has allowed effective mass human temperature screening to be carried out in a practicable and non-intrusive manner. It should not be used as an absolute temperature measurement device, but as an innovative means to conduct rapid fever screening of masses. Careful calibration of the components and proper setting of the surrounding environment are crucial in ensuring greater accuracy in the screening. Also, further health assessments by nurses must be carried out in the second tier of screening to identify suspect SARS cases.

The development of the IFss has demonstrated how Singapore's defence engineers adapted military applications and responded swiftly in the fight against the SARS virus. The success of the system was made possible only by the concerted efforts by the various parties from different government agencies and organizations. Its large-scale deployment has created positive publicity for the government's efforts in combating the virus and contributed to boosting of the degree of confidence in Singapore among both foreigners and locals.

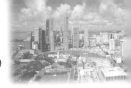

Yang How Tan

Yang How Tan is a division manager at DSTA. He leads a team of engineers responsible for development, acquisition management and operation and support of Sensor Systems for the SAF. He is a leading radar system expert in Singapore and has vast experience in sensor programme definition and development management.

The author acknowledges the contributions of DSTA members: Mr Teo Chee Wah, Mr Soo Ming Jern and Miss Evelyn Ong S C.

Contact details:
Yang How Tan
Division Manager
Sensor Systems Division
Defence Science & Technology Agency
Singapore
E-mail: tyanghow@dsta.gov.sg

Section V

Taiwan

17

Epidemiology and Control of Severe Acute Respiratory Syndrome (SARS) Outbreak in Taiwan

by *Chien-Jen Chen, Yin-Chu Chien* and *Hwai-I Yang*

Introduction

Severe acute respiratory syndrome (SARS) is a newly emerging infectious disease caused by the SARS coronavirus (SARS-CoV). The first case of SARS occurred at Guangdong, China in mid-November 2002. The local outbreak

Correspondence to: Dr. Chien-Jen Chen, Graduate Institute of Epidemiology, College of Public Health, National Taiwan University, 1 Jen-Ai Road Section 1, Taipei 10018, Taiwan. E-mail: cjchen@ha.mc.ntu.edu.tw

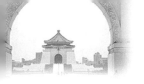

was not contained immediately and it spread from China to other countries through rapid international transportation. The disease was transmitted from an infected Chinese professor to other guests who stayed at a hotel in Hong Kong in late February. The World Health Organization (WHO) recognized SARS as a global threat in mid-March 2003, sent out an international alert and set up the SARS reporting system in mid-March. There have been 8,422 probable cases reported to the World Health Organization from 30 countries since then. The last human chain of transmission of SARS had been broken in Taiwan on 5 July 2003. During the last five months, much has been learned about the disease, including its clinical characteristics, causal agent SARS-CoV, transmission routes, and control measures. However, our knowledge about the epidemiology and ecology of SARS-CoV remains limited. There exists a distinct possibility of the resurgence of the disease. In this article, we reviewed the epidemiology and control of the SARS outbreak in Taiwan in order to provide clues for future strategies of combating the disease the next time that it strikes again.

Outbreak of SARS in Taiwan

First Cases: Period of Imported SARS

The first suspected case of SARS was reported from the National Taiwan University Hospital (NTUH) on March 10, 2003. He was a businessman who traveled to Guangdong province, China on February 5, and returned to Taipei through Hong Kong on February 21. He developed fever, myalgia and dry cough on February 25, but was not hospitalized until March 8. His wife was affected with pneumonia on March 14. By the afternoon of March 14, the couple was hospitalized in the negative-pressure isolation room of an intensive care unit (ICU) with full precautions. Their son developed fever and cough on March 17 and 20, respectively, and was hospitalized in a negative-pressure isolation room on March 21. All the three patients required mechanical ventilation. The throat swabs from the wife and son were confirmed to be associated with SARS-CoV by the reverse transcription-polymerase chain reaction (RT-PCR) test. Only one physician in the NTUH was affected with the disease.

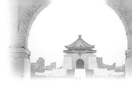

On March 26, a resident of Hong Kong's Amoy Gardens flew to Taipei and took a train to Taichung to celebrate the traditional festival, Qing Ming, with his brother. The man was treated at the China Medical University Hospital (CMUH), returned to Hong Kong, and died from SARS there. His brother was ill and treated at CMUH. He was the first case of death from SARS in Taiwan. Healthcare workers at CMUH were not affected with the disease.

As of April 14, there were 23 probable SARS cases in Taiwan. Only four of them were infected through secondary transmission, and another 19 cases were infected when they traveled to China and Hong Kong. These SARS patients were treated at different medical centers in Taiwan without inducing any hospital infection outbreak. Accurate diagnosis and immediate isolation of patients, stringent hospital infection control procedures, and quarantine of close contacts prevented the spread of the disease to family members and healthcare workers. Because of Taiwan's success in SARS control before mid-April, WHO classified Taiwan as an "area with limited local transmission".

First Outbreak: Period of Hospital Infection

Unfortunately, a large-scale outbreak of SARS infection occurred at the Taipei Municipal Hoping Hospital in mid-April. A number of healthcare workers, hospitalized patients and their relatives and visitors were infected. As there were too many SARS cases at the hospital to be treated, the hospital was closed on April 24 and patients were delivered to other hospitals in northern and southern Taiwan. The sudden closure of the hospital and relocation of patients resulted in the spread of the disease to other hospitals, including Chunghsin, Jenchi, NTUH, McKay Memorial Hospital, Yangming Hospital and Kuangdwu Hospital in Taipei; Kaohsiung Chang-Gung Memorial Hospital, Kaohsiung Medical University Hospital, and Penghu Hospital in other cities and counties. The epidemic curve of SAS had two peaks as shown in Fig. 1. The first peak was a cluster of hospital-acquired SAR patients at Taipei City in late April, while the second peak was a cluster patient at Kaohsiung City and County in mid-May.

There were 66 probable cases and 22 suspected cases reported from the outbreak at Hoping Hospital. In the outbreak at Kaohsiung Chang-Gung Memorial Hospital, 38 probable and 25 suspected cases were reported. Clusters

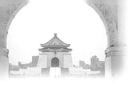

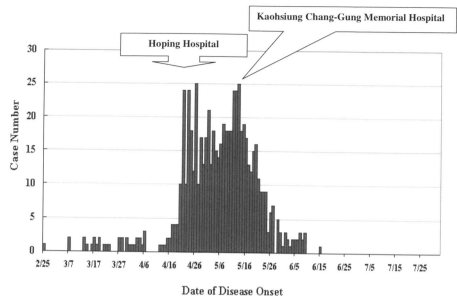

Fig. 1. Epidemic curve of SARS probable cases in Taiwan (Updated to July 31, 2003).

of SARS-affected healthcare workers found at nine additional hospitals have been linked to the initial outbreak at Hoping Hospital.

The last cluster of SARS cases occurred at Yangming Hospital at Taipei. It was the last event of hospital outbreak. The first case was an old man from a nursing home. Two affected nursing aids were considered to be the major transmission source of this outbreak. Within one day after receiving the report of cases, the entire hospital was immediately separated into two sections: one for fever patients and the other for non-fever patients. Outpatient clinics of the hospital were closed on the same day. No newly infected patient occurred ten days after the date of onset of symptoms and signs of the first SARS patient in the hospital. The last SARS case had an onset date on June 15.

During the entire period of the epidemic, the proportion of hospital-acquired infection among SARS probable cases was around 10% prior to April 22, and 90% afterward. The main reasons for the occurrence of large-scale hospital outbreaks included: (1) the failure to identify and diagnose the first SARS cases admitted to the hospitals; (2) the inadequate procedures to prevent the

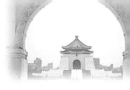

> **During the entire period of the epidemic, the proportion of hospital-acquired infection among SARS probable cases was around 10% prior to April 22, and 90% afterward.**

transmission of SARS-CoV in hospitals; (3) the poor protection of healthcare workers involved in the care of SARS patients; (4) the existence of super-spreaders; and (5) no limitation placed on the number of visitors to the hospitals or the duration of their visits.

Epidemic Characteristics

As of July 31, a total of 3,032 cases had been reported to the Center for Disease Control in Taiwan. They included 668 probable cases, 1,320 suspected cases, and 1,044 excluded cases. The incidence rate of SARS was 2.9 per 100,000 persons in Taiwan. As shown in Fig. 1, the date at the onset of symptoms and signs was February 25 for the first SARS case and June 15 for the last SARS case in Taiwan. As shown in Table 1, the period of staying in the travel alert list of WHO was 28 days for Taiwan as a whole, 41 days for Taipei, 52 days for Hong Kong and Guangdong, and 63 days for Beijing. Among the probable cases, 52 (8%) were imported from other affected regions, and 77 (12%) cases were healthcare workers.

Table 1. Period of Staying in the SARS-related Travel Alert List of World Health Organization

Area	Enlisted Date	Lifted Date	Staying Period
Beijing	April 23	June 24	63
Guangdong	April 2	May 23	52
Hong Kong	April 2	May 23	52
Taipei	May 8	June 17	41
Taiwan	May 21	June 17	28

Updated to July 31, 2003 and adopted from Taiwan CDC.

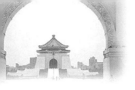

The case-fatality rate increased from zero for the group <10 years to greater than 20% for age groups between 60 and 79 years old.

As shown in Table 2, SARS affected males and females similarly. There were 52% females and 48% males in Taiwan. Most SARS cases in Taiwan were young adults. There were 434 cases (65%) aged between 20 and 59 years, and only 42 cases had ages under 20. The infection rate per 100,000 population was the lowest for the age group of under 10 years, and the highest for the age groups of 70 or more years. There were 72 probable cases who died from SARS as an underlying cause of death, thus showing an overall case-fatality rate was 11%. The case-fatality rate was higher in males (12%) than in females (9%). The case-fatality rate increased from zero for the group <10 years to greater than 20% for age groups between 60 and 79 years old. The mortality rate from SARS per 100,000 followed the same age pattern as the case fatality rate.

Table 2. Age and Gender Distribution and Fatality Rate of SARS Probable Cases in Taiwan

	No. of Cases (%)	Infection Rate (per 100,000)	No. of Cases of Death	Mortality Rate (per 100,000)	Fatality Rate (%)
Total	668	3.0	72	0.3	10.8
Gender					
Female	349 (52.2)	3.2	32	0.3	9.2
Male	319 (47.8)	2.8	40	0.3	12.5
Age (yrs)					
0–9	14 (2.1)	0.5	0	0.0	0.0
10–19	28 (4.2)	0.8	1	0.03	3.6
20–29	122 (18.3)	3.2	6	0.2	4.9
30–39	107 (16.0)	2.8	5	0.1	4.7
40–49	116 (17.4)	3.2	8	0.2	6.9
50–59	89 (13.3)	4.1	12	0.5	13.5
60–69	50 (7.5)	3.4	11	0.8	22.0
70–79	92 (13.8)	9.1	20	2.0	21.7
80+	50 (7.5)	14.2	9	2.6	18.0

Updated to July 31, 2003 and adopted from Taiwan CDC.

As shown in Table 3, the positive rate of SARS-CoV in throat swabs tested by RT-PCR for the probable, suspected, and excluded cases were 37%, 4%, and 1%, respectively. The overall positive rate of SARS-CoV was 10%. The low positive rate may be due to: (1) Some reported probable cases with symptoms and signs identical to SARS who might not be infected by SARS-CoV; (2) The RT-PCR test may not be sensitive enough to detect the virus in throat swab obtained at the early stages of the disease; and (3) Standard procedures for obtaining throat swab samples might not be followed correctly. The need is urgent to develop sensitive and specific methods for the detection of SARS-CoV at a disease stage as early as possible.

Table 4 and Fig. 2 show the geographical distribution of SARS probable cases in Taiwan. Most probable cases clustered in northern and southern Taiwan due to the large-scale hospital outbreak in these two areas. There were 520 cases (78%) in northern Taiwan, of which 462 cases (89%) were reported from Taipei City and Taipei County. The case-fatality rate was higher in southern Taiwan than in northern Taiwan.

Table 3. SARS-CoV Positive Rate of Throat Swabs from Reported SARS Cases in Taiwan

	No. of Cases A	No. of Throat Swab B	SARS Virus (+) C	Positive Rate C/B (%)
Probable	668	590	221	37.5
Suspect	1320	1036	38	3.7
Excluded	1044	911	7	0.8

Updated to July 31, 2003 and adopted from Taiwan CDC.

Table 4. Geographical Distribution of SARS Probable Cases in Taiwan

Region	No. of Probable Cases (%)	No. of Cases of Death (%)	Case Fatality Rate (%)
North	520 (77.8)	49 (68.1)	9.4
Central	36 (5.4)	2 (2.8)	5.6
South	109 (16.3)	20 (27.8)	18.3
East	3 (0.5)	1 (1.4)	33.3
Total	668	72	10.8

Updated to July 31, 2003 adopted from Taiwan CDC.

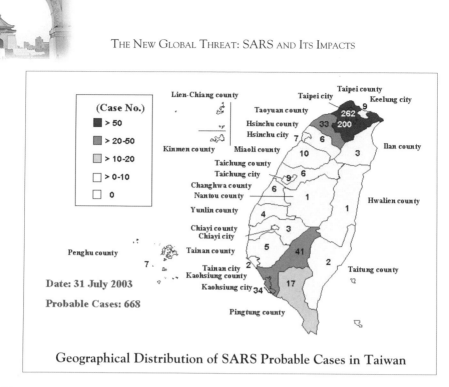

Geographical Distribution of SARS Probable Cases in Taiwan

Fig. 2. Numbers of SARS probable cases by city and county in Taiwan (updated to July 31, 2003).

SARS Control Strategies in Taiwan

The Taiwan government has taken a number of measures to control the spread of SARS, including the organization of a SARS advisory committee, isolation treatment of reported cases, infection-control training, contact tracing and quarantine, hospital infection surveillance, and airport and seaport surveillance. An Inter-ministry Committee was established to coordinate these efforts through central-local and international collaboration.

SARS Advisory Committee and National SARS Control and Mitigation Committee

The Department of Health set up a SARS Advisory Committee in mid-March. It comprised epidemiologists, clinical physicians, virologists and infectious

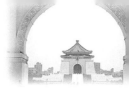

disease specialists. The committee was set up to review daily reported SARS cases, to ensure the transparency of the epidemic information, to update knowledge and experiences of SARS containment, and to provide suggestions for any strategies taken by the government and the public to control the disease.

After the outbreak of SARS in Hoping Hospital at Taipei, a National SARS Control and Mitigation Committee was established by the Executive Yuan on April 28, 2003. The Prime Minister chaired the committee with the all ministers of the Executive Yuan as members. A special law was approved by the Legislative Yuan to promote the control and mitigation of SARS in Taiwan. A special budget of NT$50 billions was allocated to the program.

SARS Control Strategies

Several strategies for the prevention and intervention of the SARS outbreak have been implemented. They included: (1) Health education on prevention, early detection, prompt reporting and treatment of SARS via posters, mass media, brochures and websites (started on March 20); (2) Ten-days home quarantine for passengers coming from SARS-affected areas and all contacts of reported SARS cases (started on March 27; (3) Classification of SARS as a Class-4 notifiable communicable disease in order to reinforce the control activities implemented by the government on March 28; (4) Airport/seaport surveillance of in- and out-bound passengers for screening and banning of any imported and exported SARS cases through SARS questionnaire interviews (started on March 29); (5) Body temperature monitoring and distribution of guidelines on standard procedures for SARS prevention and reporting, for all arriving and departing passengers from April 10 to June 2; (6) Isolation of all staff and patients of the Hoping Hospital on April 24; (7) Strengthening the control of hospital-acquired infection in all hospitals; (8) Isolation of residents of Huachang civil building in Taipei City on May 9; (9) SARS prevention TV programs broadcast daily at regular hours to announce governmental measures and policies on SARS control from May 6 to June 15; (10) A national campaign of temperature-measuring to check for fever, with a fever hotline set up by the Taiwan Medical Association for professional counseling on the SARS control; and (11) Setting-up of 195 fever-screening stations to seek out fever subjects on June 1.

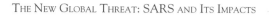

International cooperation has been proved to be an important key determinant in the fight against SARS in the "earth village".

Laboratory Tests of SARS-CoV

Additionally, laboratory diagnosis of SARS-CoV was set up quickly in Taiwan. The first strain of SARS-CoV was cultured in Vero-E6 on April 9. On the end of May, 11 strains of SARS-CoV had been cultured and sequenced for the full 29,714 nucleotides for each strain in Taiwan. These findings were helpful in order to understand the source of the SARS epidemic in Taiwan and improve the ability of SARS differentiation. SARS research has been included in the national genomic and medical technology program for the improvement of knowledge in this new emerging disease.

International Collaboration

International cooperation has been proved to be an important key determinant in the fight against SARS in the "earth village". Experts from the US CDC and WHO have helped Taiwan in the control of SARS. In collaboration with Taiwan CDC, they improved the SARS reporting system, the standard protocol for epidemiological investigation, the inspection of infection control programs in various hospitals, and the establishment and quality assurance of laboratory examinations.

There is no national boundary for SARS. No nation may be left out the global outbreak alert and response network without breaking the security for all people in the world. In order to properly fulfill our role in global health, Taiwan reported the epidemic situation to the WHO as soon as SARS cases were detected in mid-March. Taiwan also hosted an international symposium on SARS epidemic on April 20 and 21. In addition, Taiwan ensures that all information is correct and transparent. We also try our best to help the international community to understand our efforts on SARS control and share Taiwan's experiences with others.

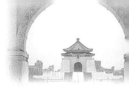

SARS would not be the last emerging communicable disease, and we will continue to face challenges from unknown diseases in the future.

Future Perspectives

SARS would not be the last emerging communicable disease, and we will continue to face challenges from unknown diseases in the future. As lessons we have been learned from the SARS outbreak, we shall continue to upgrade and improve the capacity of the "Emerging Infectious Disease Reporting System". Fever-screening stations and airport/seaport surveillance of passengers will be maintained to seek out fever subjects at the first contact. Measures to control hospital-acquired infection in all hospitals will continue to be strengthened. A rapid and precise method of SARS-CoV diagnosis is under vigorous research and development. A databank and inventorized biospecimens of SARS cases are being established. The coverage rate of influenza vaccination will be promoted in autumn and winter, especially among the elderly, healthcare workers, and subjects with chronic diseases. Inter-ministry collaboration and international cooperation will also be strengthened.

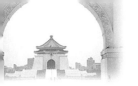

CHIEN-JEN CHEN

Dr. Chien-jen Chen is Minister, Department of Health, Executive Yuan, Republic of China, Taipei (May 2003–Present); Vice Chairman, National Science Council, Taipei; Professor, Graduate Institute of Epidemiology, National Taiwan University School of Public Health; Senior Associate, Department of Epidemiology, Johns Hopkins University School of Hygiene and Public Health, Baltimore; and Adjunct Professor, Department of Biostatistics and Epidemiology, Tulane University, New Orleans.

Dr. Chen obtained his M.P.H. degree from the National Taiwan University, Taipei, Taiwan (1975); and his Sc.D. degree from the Johns Hopkins University, Baltimore, USA (1982) (majored in Epidemiology and Human Genetics).

Honors, Awards And Prizes

Among his numerous honors and awards are:

President Award, National Taiwan University (1970)

Outstanding Youth Award, Chinese Youth Corps (1973)

Outstanding Research Award, National Science Council, ROC (1986–1996)

Fogarty International Research Fellowship Award, US National Institute of Health (1989)

Outstanding Teaching Award, Ministry of Education, ROC (1992)

Fellow, American College of Epidemiology, USA (1993)

Outstanding Scholar, Foundation for the Advancement of Outstanding Scholarship (1995–1999)

Health Medal, Department of Health, ROC (1996)

Academician, Academia Sinica (1998)

Outstanding Anti-Cancer Research Award, Taiwan Cancer Foundation (1999)

National Chair Professor, Ministry of Education, ROC (1999–2002)

ISI Citation Classic Award, ISI Thomas Scientific (2001)

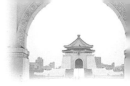

Some Representative Publications

Chen C.J., Chuang Y.C., Lin T.M. and Wu H.Y. Malignant neoplasms among residents of a blackfoot disease-endemic area in Taiwan: High-arsenic artesian well water and cancers. *Cancer Res.* 45: 5895–5899, 1985.

Chen C.J., Wu M.M., Lee S.S., Wang J.D., Cheng S.H. and Wu H.Y. Atherogenicity and carcinogenicity of high-arsenic artesian well water: Multiple risk factors and related malignant neoplasms of blackfoot disease. *Arteriosclerosis* 8: 452–460, 1988.

Chen C.J., Kuo T.L. and Wu M.M. Arsenic and cancers. *Lancet* 1: 414–415, 1988.

Chen C.J. and Wang C.J. 1990. Ecological correlation between arsenic level in well water and age-adjusted mortality from malignant neoplasms. *Cancer Res.* 50: 5470–5474.

Chen C.J. Blackfoot disease. *Lancet* 336: 442, 1990.

Chen C.J., Liang K.Y., Chang A.S., Chang Y.C., Lu S.N., Liaw Y.F., Chang W.Y., Sheen M.C. and Lin T.M. Effects of hepatitis B virus, alcohol drinking, cigarette smoking and familial tendency on hepatocellular carcinoma. *Hepatology* 13: 398–406, 1991.

Chen C.J., Chen C.W., Wu M.M. and Kuo T.L. Cancer potential in liver, lung, bladder and kidney due to ingested inorganic arsenic in drinking water. *Br. J. Cancer* 66: 888–892, 1992.

Chen C.J., Hsueh Y.M., Lai M.S., Hsu M.P., Wu M.M. and Tai T.Y. Increased prevalence of hypertension and long-term arsenic exposure. *Hypertension* 25: 53–60, 1995.

Chen C.J., Chiou H.Y. and Chiang M.H. Dose-response relationship between ischemic heart disease mortality and long-term arsenic exposure. *Arterioslcer. Thrombo. Vasc. Biol.* 16:504–510, 1996.

Chen C.J., Yu M.W., Liaw Y.F., Wang L.W., Chiamprasert S., Matin F., Hirvonen A., Bell A.B. and Santella R.M. Chronic hepatitis B carriers with null genotypes of glutathione S-transferase M1 and T1 polymorphisms who are exposed to aflatoxins are at increased risk of hepatocellular carcinoma. *Am. J. Hum. Genet.* 59: 128–134, 1996.

Chen C.J., Wang L.Y., Lu S.N., Wu M.H., You S.L., Li H.P., Zhang Y.J., Wang L.W. and Santella R.M. Elevated aflatoxin exposure and increased risk of hepatocellular carcinoma. *Hepatology* 24: 38–42, 1996.

Chang M.H., Chen C.J., Lai M.S., Kong M.S., Wu T.C., Liang D.C., Hsu H.M., Shau W.Y. and Chen D.S. Taiwan Childhood Hepatoma Study Group. 1997. Nationwide hepatitis B vaccination and the incidence of hepatocellular carcinoma in children in Taiwan. *N. Engl. J. Med.* 336: 1855–1859.

Section VI

Toronto

18

SARS in Canada: The Story of SARS in Canada is Essentially Toronto's Tale

by *Pauline Chan*

SARS came to Canada on a flight from Hong Kong in late February 2003. 78-year-old Sui-chu Kwan and her 79-year-old husband had spent 10 days in Hong Kong on what should have been a treasured vacation. For most of their visit, the elderly Toronto couple stayed with family and friends but they allowed themselves one indulgence. It would prove to be a deadly one.

The two were offered a night's stay at one of a number of nicely-appointed hotels. They chose Kowloon's Metropole Hotel, and were placed on the ninth floor. It was the same floor where a 64-year-old physician from China was staying. The doctor had been in Guangdong province, treating patients suffering from a mysterious atypical pneumonia. It's believed the Kwans picked up SARS through contact with this man.

Correspondence to: Pauline Chan, CFTO News, Canada; E-mail: pchan@ctv.ca

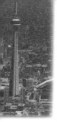

Ironically, a Vancouver man was also exposed to SARS at the Metropole Hotel. He would return to his home on Canada's west coast around the same time as Kwan's son would be admitted to a Toronto hospital with severe respiratory distress. But the Toronto experience with SARS somehow proved to be vastly different from that in Vancouver.

In Toronto, Sui-chu Kwan became ill shortly after her return from vacation on February 23. She fell into a coma and died on March 5 without ever being treated in hospital. Her body was taken directly to the funeral home and health officials were informed she had a history of high blood pressure as well as a recent bout of influenza. Her cause of death was given as "heart attack".

On March 7, Kwan's son Chi Kwai Tse was brought by ambulance to Scarborough Grace Hospital in east Toronto. The emergency room was typically overcrowded. The nurse who treated Tse that evening, noted he had a fever and cough. No doubt he believed he had picked up the same chest infection that his mother and father had developed after their Hong Kong vacation. In total, 6 members of the Kwan family would pick up SARS. The disease would claim two lives — Sui-chu Kwan and her son Chi Kwai Tse.

While Mrs. Kwan was Toronto's Patient Zero, it was her son who set off an explosive series of medical events.

While in hospital, Chi Kwai Tse was kept in an observation area. Just a couple of meters away was the bed of 76-year-old Joseph Pollack, who was being examined for an apparent heart ailment. Between the two men was a simple cloth curtain. Also in the room was a 77-year old man, who apparently also contracted SARS. He died two weeks later, but not before passing on the illness to others. Pollack also picked up the virus, continuing the chain of transmission.

Tse's case eventually sparked an astonishing numbers of others — in relatives, health workers, other patients, hospital visitors. Chi Kwai Tse died March 13, still undiagnosed. Joseph Pollack was sent home, thinking that his health was once again assured, after dealing with his cardiac troubles. He would infect his wife and returned to Scarborough Grace Hospital on March 16 with the characteristic high fever associated with SARS. As hospital staff dealt with Joseph Pollack, his wife Rose, sat in the emergency waiting room with other patients, among them, a Filipino man with a leg ailment, accompanied by his two sons. Their contact with Rose Pollack would set off another set of infections and hundreds of quarantines.

From mid-March onwards, SARS became the all-absorbing topic for hospitals and public officials.

It was not until March 14, that Toronto Public Health officials held an evening news conference to alert the public about what was then identified only as "atypical pneumonia". They described the symptoms as "sudden fever, coughing, shortness of breath…" and they urged anyone who had recent contact with Siu-chu Kwan or her son Chi Kwai Tse to contact medical authorities. Three hospitals were identified as places where the victims had sought treatment and where transmission of the mysterious illness could have occurred: Scarborough Grace, Mount Sinai and Sunnybrook and Women's College Hospital. An information hotline was also set up. In the three months following that announcement, SARS became a daily fixture in the newspapers and broadcasts. Since healthcare in Canada generally comes under provincial jurisdiction, a combination of Toronto and Ontario officials worked together to deal with the crisis.

In hindsight, Toronto health officials can compare their experiences with those of their counterparts in Vancouver, where a 55-year-old man returned from Hong Kong already showing signs of illness. He had also stayed at the Metropole Hotel. The man was quickly isolated and recovered, without sparking a search for contacts in the community or widespread quarantines. His connection with the Far East gave doctors a far better clue to track down the cause of his illness than Toronto's first SARS patient, who arrived in hospital with no obvious connection to Hong Kong and believing that his mother had died of a heart attack at home.

From mid-March onwards, SARS became the all-absorbing topic for hospitals and public officials. On March 26, Ontario Premier Ernie Eves declared SARS a provincial emergency. The elderly Filipino man, who was at Scarborough Grace Hospital with Rose Pollack, died April 1, apparently of SARS, presumably contracted during his wait in the emergency waiting room or perhaps from infected staff. His sons left the hospital to continue their regular activities, including meetings with a charismatic religious group called "Bukas Loob sa Dios", or BLD. The international organization boasted 500 members in the Toronto area. Their meeting center was a west end church,

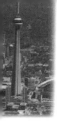

Our Lady of the Assumption. Two weeks later, several members of the group began showing signs of respiratory illness; some 30 people, including three children were suspected of having SARS. As a result, all 500 members of the Toronto BLD group were voluntarily quarantined. Fortunately, health officials were able to contact all individuals involved and isolation was not a problem.

Of the thousands of quarantine cases during Toronto's SARS outbreak, voluntary confinement was only a problem in a couple of cases. In early April, an employee of Hewlett-Packard in Markham, just north of Toronto, failed to observe his full 10-day quarantine. He returned to work early but began to show symptoms soon after, prompting the quarantine of 197 co-workers on April 10. The 62-year-old man subsequently died on May 24, the 25th victim of SARS in the province. Health officials also expressed public concern about a doctor who ignored SARS symptoms and attended a funeral on April 18 and church services the following day. The unidentified man became belligerent when ordered into quarantine. Although health officials speculated about what range of measures they would or could take to force a non-compliant individual into isolation, no further action was required in this or any other cases. The resident of York Region was hospitalized and co-operated fully with public health staff thereafter.

By April 19, SARS deaths in the Greater Toronto area numbered 14. Most of those affected by SARS remained nameless through the weeks of daily updates listing numbers of people quarantined, probable cases, suspect cases and deaths. But one highly visible patient came from the ranks of the medical staff researching the disease. Dr. Allison McGeer is the Director of Infectious Disease Control at Mount Sinai Hospital and is one of Canada's leading experts on the topic. She contracted SARS while researching the disease at Scarborough Grace Hospital, in the early stages of the outbreak.

Her infection also prompted the quarantine of several key research figures, including Dr. Donald Low. Dr. Low was arguably the foremost spokesperson in the city's daily SARS news conferences, seeking to inform the public about the latest developments, combat further spread of the disease and reassure the city. He appeared regularly alongside Dr. Sheela Basrur, Toronto's Medical Officer of Health, Dr James Young, who bears the twin hats of Ontario's Commissioner of Public Safety and Security, as well as Ontario's Chief Coroner, and Dr. Colin D'Cunha, Ontario's Commissioner of Public Health. The fact that two prominent physicians, Dr. McGeer and Dr. Low, were

knocked out of the mix by the very disease on which they were supposed to be authorities, added to the fears of the general public and medical workers.

At the same time, several Toronto area hospitals were also struggling with staff shortages due to illness and quarantines. Not only were Scarborough Grace, Mount Sinai and Sunnybrook closed to new patients while under quarantine early in the outbreak, but other hospitals, such as North York General, Toronto General, York Central Hospital also experienced partial closures. Those affected included expectant mothers, emergency cases and those awaiting diagnostic tests. Other hospitals had to pick up the slack and ambulances were re-routed. Stress levels for medical staff soared, as did public concern about who would be available to treat Toronto's 2.5 million residents (5 million in the Greater Toronto Area), should they fall ill.

Facilities dedicated to SARS diagnosis opened across the Toronto area. The first so-called "SARS Assessment Centre" opened March 27 at Women's College Hospital in the downtown core. Throughout the first week of April, other specialized facilities opened in Markham, Etobicoke, Scarborough and Oshawa, ensuring coverage for the Greater Toronto region.

At this point, some 66 healthcare workers had been infected and the government began to loosen its purse strings in an effort to ease the burden on hospitals. On April 22, Provincial Health Minister Tony Clement announced 2.5 million dollars in funding for SARS research as well as detailing the "New Normal": heightened safety and hygiene recommendations for all. Doubling surgical gloves, doubling surgical gowns, eye protection, N-95 masks (which were already in short supply as members of the public stocked up) were all to be part of the "New Normal". Instructions on proper hand-washing were issued, broadcast and posted. Sales of alcohol, anti-bacterial soaps, handy wipes, even tissues, jumped. Pearson International Airport installed thermal scanners to check air passengers for fevers while questionnaires to screen for

On April 22, Provincial Health Minister Tony Clement announced 2.5 million dollars in funding for SARS research as well as detailing the "New Normal": heightened safety and hygiene recommendations for all.

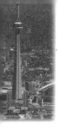

SARS were handed out in numerous settings including the airport, schools, nursing homes and health clinics.

Other adjustments made in the community included changes in religious practices. Easter Sunday fell on April 20, which meant that preparations for the most solemn feast in the Christian calendar were being made in early April, at the height of the SARS outbreak. Churches made public announcements supporting the containment efforts of the Public Health Department. As a result, containers of Holy water, in which Catholics traditionally dip their hands upon entering a Church, were left dry. Communion which is usually placed either in the hand or on the tongue of the communicant, was offered only on the hands. The serving of sacramental wine, usually offered in a communal cup, was debated, with some churches opting to eliminate wine offered to the congregation. Hand shaking, a greeting practiced as part of the weekly Catholic service, and the kissing of a crucifix, part of Easter services, were modified to minimize person-to-person contact. Orthodox services, conducted two weeks later, were the subject of similar discussions but most of their Easter services were conducted according to tradition.

A graph of probable SARS cases on the Health Canada website shows that infections were tailing off by the third week of April. Out of 137 probable cases, the vast number occurred in healthcare settings, five were listed as travel-related and the rest, either via familial connections or within the BLD religious group (six cases). None had occurred as a result of general activity within the community. All cases could be traced and healthcare officials believed the outbreak was under control and nearing the end, which is why an announcement by the World Health Organization on April 23 stung public officials and residents so much.

On April 23, Toronto became the first city outside of Asia to come under a travel advisory. On April 2, the WHO issued its first travel advisory, recommending travelers postpone visits to Hong Kong because of SARS. The extension of the advisory to Toronto was made at the same time as Beijing and Shanxi Province in China, where the number of infections and fatalities vastly outnumbered those in Canada (15 deaths at the time, 261 probable and suspected cases). Dr. David Heymann, the WHO's Executive Director of Communicable Diseases, warned the advisory would remain in place for a minimum of three weeks, twice the maximum incubation period for SARS.

SARS had already had a devastating impact on Toronto's economy from late March.

A flurry of activity ensued on the part of Canadian health and government agencies. A party flew to Geneva to try and lift the advisory. Discussions between Canadian and WHO authorities were carried out swiftly and the WHO did remove the travel advisory just six days later, on April 29, after determining that the outbreak was contained and screening of air travelers would minimize the risk of exporting SARS. But significant damage was already done. SARS had already had a devastating impact on Toronto's economy from late March and the stifling effects of a travel edict from such a highly regarded agency as the World Health Organization would last well beyond six days.

Although Canada has an image of being a winter destination, summer is the time when Toronto is at its busiest, especially for the tourism industry. Major events include Caribana, the Molson Indy, the DuMaurier Jazz Festival, Gay Pride Week and the Canadian National Exhibition. But during the travel advisory, conventions were cancelled and movie stars such as Halle Berry avoided the city often called "Hollywood North", citing concerns about SARS. Even baseball players were advised not to sign autographs although they did continue to play professional games. School trips to Toronto from abroad, especially the United States, were cancelled and students and athletes from Toronto were made unwelcome in other places, jeopardizing the college prospects of young Canadians hoping to win sports scholarships in American universities. Hotels, which usually boasted 80–90 per cent occupancy during the summer, were down to 40 or even 30 per cent. Business was cut in half for taxis, certain retailers and entertainment venues such as live theatre performances and other attractions. Chinese stores and restaurants in the city were already hit hard by misplaced public concerns early on in the SARS outbreak and grew increasingly alarmed with the issuing of the WHO advisory.

The city responded with a range of initiatives to revive its economy and especially tourism. Air travelers were greeted with small gifts packages containing free items and coupons, some even being handed out by the Mayor himself. A promotional campaign was launched called "Time for a Little T.O.", offering a discount deal for tickets to either Disney's "The Lion King" or the

At the height of "SARS Two", some 5000 people were under voluntary quarantine.

musical "Mamma Mia" plus baseball tickets and dinner at certain participating restaurants. These packages were snapped up, largely by Southern Ontario residents. "I Love TO" T-shirts were designed and sold. Video campaigns were beamed via satellite to the international community. The federal government promised 100 million dollars for the city's SARS recovery efforts, along with 118 million dollars pledged by the provincial government. Politicians, including Prime Minister Jean Chretien, made a point of dining at Chinese restaurants while posing for news cameras. And celebrities, particularly Canadians, were enlisted to sing the city's praises globally. Mike Meyers, Shania Twain, even the Rolling Stones voiced their support for Toronto.

While the city remained on WHO's list of SARS affected areas until May 14, it breathed a massive sigh of relief at the lifting of the advisory on April 29. While it recognized that the economic harm done by SARS would take weeks, maybe months to repair, it was confident that it had turned the corner in the fight against the disease.

That confidence would be shaken, however, with a second wave of SARS, which began nearly a month later. Toronto feared a second travel advisory would sound the death knell for many businesses, already brought to the brink of financial ruin. The source of the second round of infections is believed to be a man in his 90's who was treated at North York General. Like the majority of Toronto's SARS fatalities, he had several underlying illnesses which hampered diagnosis. He likely became exposed to SARS while in a hospital setting and he died on May 22. As of mid-July, Health Canada lists all of the probable cases of SARS in the second wave as traced to healthcare or familial settings.

At the height of "SARS Two", some 5000 people were under voluntary quarantine. Staff at North York General, Scarborough General and St. John's Rehabilitation Centre were placed under a "working quarantine", instituted to avoid a situation in which so many healthcare workers might be at home under quarantine that the hospitals and ambulance service might not be able to function at all. The frontline healthcare workers would be isolated from their families while at home but still report to work using full safety precautions.

Still, one of those workers would become Canada's first healthcare worker to die of SARS.

Nelia Laroza, a 51-year-old orthopedic nurse at North York General, fell ill in mid-May and died on June 29. She was the 39th victim of the disease. Her 16-year-old son, Kenneth, began showing symptoms at the end of May, causing the closure of his school, Father Michael McGivney Catholic Academy in Markham on May 28. It re-opened after completing a 10-day quarantine.

Laroza's funeral on July 4 was attended by Ontario Premier Ernie Eves, Health Minister Tony Clement, and an emotional Chief Coroner Dr. James Young. There was also an honor guard of fellow nurses and emergency services personnel and hundreds of others, all paying tribute to Laroza as well as all frontline medical staff. The sentiments were similar to those expressed after the terrorist attacks of September 11, with the eyes of a nation, or at least a community, opened to the dangers faced by medical workers. Appreciation and respect for doctors, nurses and paramedics who regularly risked their health and very lives for others was dramatically heightened. Figures such as Toronto's Medical Officer of Health, Dr. Sheela Basrur, and microbiologist Dr. Donald Low of Mount Sinai Hospital are now regularly greeted with applause and congratulations at public ceremonies, with some members of the public even seeking to have their pictures taken with the new healthcare superstars.

By the end of June, the cost of fighting the disease, according to provincial health officials, stood at 945-million dollars and counting. Infections were tapering off and attention once again focused on helping the city's economic recovery with a series of large public events. A televised ceremony honoring several Canadians with stars on Toronto's Walk of Fame was held on June 25. Singer Shania Twain, actor Mike Myers and model Linda Evangelista and others put their glamor and celebrity on stage to show support for the city. Toronto's Molson Indy on the July 5-6 weekend was well-attended and to add to the positive atmosphere, the race was won by hometown boy, Paul Tracy.

By the end of June, the cost of fighting the disease, according to provincial health officials, stood at 945-million dollars and counting.

Attendance at Toronto's Gay Pride week at the end of June was bolstered by the fact that the Ontario court had just issued a ruling essentially legalizing gay marriages in the province, prompting many out of town visitors to make wedding plans while attending events at the 23rd annual gay and lesbian festival. Traditionally, it is one of the three largest gay/lesbian festivals in the world, attracting up to a million people to its final parade and pumping 74-million dollars into the local economy in 2002. Many Toronto businesses are resigned to the fact that profits for summer 2003 will not live up to expectations but, with help from various publicity campaigns, they hope to mend Toronto's image enough to assure future viability.

At the time of this writing, Toronto is anticipating the start of Caribana, held in the week leading up to Ontario's civic holiday on August 4. The annual celebration of Toronto's Caribbean community also attracts up to a million people for its spectacular costumed parade, with many visitors coming in from the United States, the Caribbean and Britain.

One event planned specifically for Toronto's SARS recovery was a concert featuring Canadian pop stars. The June 21st show, headlined by Sarah McLaughlan, the Tragically Hip, Diana Krall, Our Lady Peace, the Barenaked Ladies and Avril Lavigne was held at two venues simultaneously, the Air Canada Centre and Skydome. Seventy-thousand music fans attended but that event will be dwarfed by another concert which promises to be the highlight of Toronto's summer.

The Rolling Stones are set to play a benefit for Toronto on July 30. The venue is Downsview Park, a former military base and the site of last year's World Youth Day papal mass and vigil. 800-thousand young Catholics from around the world attended the event in late July 2002. Officials for the SARS benefit plan to cap attendance at 600-thousand. Ticket sales, at the bargain price of $21.50 Cdn., have gone well with 420-thousand sold, just over a week before the show. Sixty-thousand tickets were sold to U.S. residents.

In early May, federal politician Dennis Mills initiated efforts to approach the Rolling Stones in the middle of a world tour because of their high profile and their well-known fondness for Toronto. They had used the city in the past as a home base to prepare for other concert tours. After receiving a favorable initial response from the band, efforts were made to arrange the 10-million dollars in funding, required to set up the concert. Other big names

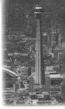

such as AC/DC, Justin Timberlake and Canadian rockers Rush were later added to the bill.

It may seem curious that so much emphasis has been placed on a group of high profile musicians in the midst of a medical crisis. But if Public Health officials can be transformed into pseudo-celebrities by Toronto's SARS experiences, perhaps a band of rock stars can play a key role in restoring the city's economic health. In the two weeks leading up to the Downsview concert, another nurse had died of SARS, a 58-year-old woman who worked at the William Osler Health Centre in Toronto's west end. She was the 41st SARS victim in Ontario.

While the economic effects of SARS were swift and harsh, Toronto retailers and other businesses are optimistic that the losses of summer 2003 will be replaced by business as usual in the fall. What will likely be a more lasting legacy of SARS will be a new focus on public health. The new "hero" status accorded to healthcare workers will be an important tool as Toronto and Ontario seek more funding for healthcare in the coming months and years. Toronto's SARS experiences have highlighted the need for more doctors and nurses, particularly in the public health field. Currently, there are only five physicians in the city's Public Health Department. Officials in the department also cite the need for improved communications, especially with hospitals. And as Dr. Bonnie Henry, Toronto's Associate Medical Officer of Health, points out, flu season is coming up in the fall. Medical staff will have to deal with heightened public sensitivity to respiratory symptoms. No doubt patients will be more prompt and more insistent about seeking a physician's attention than in previous years. Increased anxiety and general fatigue among healthcare workers will also put extra strain on the system. In addition to the scores of healthcare workers who were infected themselves, other nurses and physicians worked long and hard from March to July and are exhausted from treating SARS patients. Politicians and physicians will have to seize the moment to ensure that resources are put into these areas while the experiences of summer 2003 are fresh in everyone's mind.